Cardiac Catheterization:
An Atlas and DVD

Cardiac Catheterization:
An Atlas and DVD

Michael Ragosta, MD, FACC
Associate Professor of Medicine
Director, Cardiac Catheterization Laboratories
University of Virginia Health System
Charlottesville, Virginia

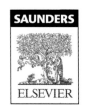

SAUNDERS

ELSEVIER

SAUNDERS
ELSEVIER

1600 John F. Kennedy Blvd.
Ste 1800
Philadelphia, PA 19103-2899

CARDIAC CATHETERIZATION: AN ATLAS AND DVD   ISBN: 978-1-4160-3999-0

Library of Congress Cataloging-in-Publication Data

Ragosta, Michael.
 Cardiac catheterization : an atlas and DVD / Michael Ragosta. -- 1st ed.
   p. ; cm.
 Includes bibliographical references and index.
 ISBN 978-1-4160-3999-0
 1. Cardiac catheterization--Atlases. I. Title.
 [DNLM: 1. Heart Catheterization--Atlases. WG 17 R144c 2010]
 RC683.5.C25R34 2010
 616.1'207540222--dc22

                                                 2009002449

Acquisitions Editor: Natasha Andjelkovic
Project Manager: Mary Stermel
Design Direction: Steve Stave
Marketing Manager: Courtney Ingram

Printed in China

Last digit is the print number: 9 8 7 6 5 4 3 2 1

CONTENTS

PREFACE

Cardiac catheterization laboratories are very exciting places. Lives are routinely saved in this fast-paced, high-tech environment, and even the most jaded clinicians find the diagnostic and therapeutic procedures fascinating. In addition to clinical service, other functions vital to a modern hospital, such as education, training, and clinical research, are centered in the cardiac catheterization laboratory.

Percutaneous interventional procedures often receive greater interest than the less glamorous, invasive diagnostic studies. However, the fundamental skills inherent to diagnostic catheterization form the foundation for more complicated procedures. It is crucial that an operator become highly proficient in the techniques used to gain arterial and venous access, enter the various chambers of the heart, measure and interpret hemodynamic waveforms, and perform and interpret angiography of the heart chambers, the coronary arteries, and the aorta and its branches.

In addition to mastering the physical manipulations required to perform cardiac catheterization, a competent clinician must also learn to carefully scrutinize the angiographic and physiologic data produced during the procedure. There is a disturbing tendency to equate procedural speed with technical proficiency. While an efficiently performed procedure is desirable, the operator has failed if the end result of this frantic effort is a collection of nondiagnostic images and indecipherable data. There is simply no excuse for poor-quality angiograms and sloppy hemodynamic studies, and it goes without saying that the capable clinician always strives to obtain the highest-quality diagnostic data.

Finally, in addition to technical proficiency and production of high-quality data, competency entails a solid understanding of the array of normal and pathologic findings and the ability to recognize and manage all potential complications.

It is the goal of this book to help the operator master these fundamental skills. All routinely performed diagnostic catheterization procedures are described in detail, emphasizing the practical and technical aspects of the techniques. Importantly, this book is designed to serve as an image atlas. Still frames in the text are augmented by almost 200 movies contained on the enclosed DVD representative of both common and rare conditions encountered during diagnostic catheterization. This book attempts to distill many years of experience into a single volume with the inclusion of images collected over 15 years of practice in a busy, cardiac catheterization laboratory.

This book and supplemental DVD are designed primarily for cardiologists in training, practicing cardiologists, and cardiac catheterization laboratory nurses and technicians. Both novice and advanced individuals will find interest in the text and in the wide breadth of images available for review. The book and supplemental DVD may also be of interest to anyone involved in the care of cardiac patients, including coronary care unit nurses, nurse practitioners, physician assistants, and internal medicine and critical care physicians.

"To study the phenomenon of disease without books is to sail an uncharted sea, while to study books without patients is not to go to sea at all."

Sir William Osler

ACKNOWLEDGMENTS

The abundant examples of normal and pathologic conditions observed in the cardiac catheterization laboratory form the core of this book and atlas. These could not have been collected single-handedly. Aware of my obsession with finding the perfect example of each of these entities, I would like to thank my colleagues, namely Drs. Ian J. Sarembock, Eric R. Powers, Scott D. Lim, and Lawrence W. Gimple, as well as many of the cardiology fellows at the University of Virginia for their ongoing vigilance for the ideal "teaching case." Their contributions augmented my teaching collection and provided many of the cases appearing in this work. I would also like to pay tribute to the many patients I had the privilege of caring for and whose images are provided here. All physicians recognize that one never wants to be inflicted with an "interesting disease"; I hope there is some consolation to the patients included in this work that their afflictions offer valuable lessons, thereby helping future patients. Finally, I want to thank my wife, Kiyoko, and my three marvelous children, Nick, Tony, and Sachi, for their support and patience while writing this text.

PATIENT EVALUATION

Many functions vital to modern medical centers occur in the cardiac catheterization laboratory. Cardiologists perform numerous diagnostic and life-saving therapeutic procedures each day in this highly technical environment. Countless physicians, nurses, and technicians regularly undergo important medical training, and many of the recent strides in cardiovascular medicine are based on research activities focused in the cardiac catheterization laboratory.

The complex and fast-paced environment that characterizes the modern cardiac catheterization laboratory also provides an ideal breeding ground for serious problems. Catheter-based procedures entail significant patient risks, and the consequences of even minor mistakes can be devastating. Ensuring that each patient undergoes proper evaluation before catheterization and that the appropriate procedures are performed with the minimal possible risk are important principles that underlie all successful cardiac catheterization laboratory enterprises. Importantly, optimal patient outcomes depend on a "systems"-based approach with development of patient care protocols based on input and cooperation of a team of professionals including physicians, nurses, pharmacists, technicians, and administrators.

Preprocedural Evaluation. All patients require a thorough evaluation before undergoing a procedure in the catheterization laboratory consisting of a focused history and physical examination, and a review of pertinent tests such as laboratory values, the electrocardiogram, noninvasive studies, and prior catheterizations.

Table 1-1 lists the crucial elements in the patient's medical history. It is important to screen for any history of bleeding or recent surgery that may influence the use of heparin, aspirin, or platelet inhibitors. Similarly, several comorbid conditions such as renal failure, pulmonary, cerebrovascular, and peripheral vascular disease are predictive of increased risk of catheterization and impact decisions regarding surgical versus percutaneous revascularization. Details of prior peripheral vascular surgery or intervention are important to determine the route of arterial access chosen for catheterization. This must be defined before the procedure and not when the operator is finding it difficult to secure vascular access. For patients who have undergone prior coronary bypass surgery, it is imperative to know the nature and location of the bypass grafts. Similarly, it is helpful to review the angiograms of patients who have undergone a previous cardiac catheterization or coronary intervention. Other important issues to discern include the presence of a patient's advanced directives and "do not resuscitate" orders, blood product refusal, the patient's ability to follow directions, communicate, and give informed consent, and for female patients, their childbearing potential and the need for pregnancy testing before the procedure.

A precatheterization physical examination focuses on the cardiovascular system. Auscultation of the heart assesses for the presence of murmurs. Examination of the brachial, radial, femoral, and distal lower extremity pulses is critical to determine the location of arterial access. In addition to palpation, the examiner should auscultate over the femoral, abdominal, and subclavian areas in search of bruits that might suggest the presence of occlusive disease. Blood

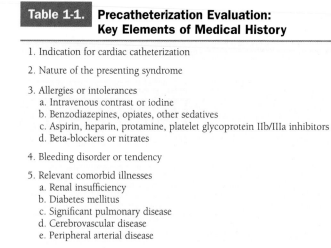

Table 1-1. **Precatheterization Evaluation: Key Elements of Medical History**

1. Indication for cardiac catheterization

2. Nature of the presenting syndrome

3. Allergies or intolerances
   a. Intravenous contrast or iodine
   b. Benzodiazepines, opiates, other sedatives
   c. Aspirin, heparin, protamine, platelet glycoprotein IIb/IIIa inhibitors
   d. Beta-blockers or nitrates

4. Bleeding disorder or tendency

5. Relevant comorbid illnesses
   a. Renal insufficiency
   b. Diabetes mellitus
   c. Significant pulmonary disease
   d. Cerebrovascular disease
   e. Peripheral arterial disease

6. Prior coronary diagnostic or revascularization procedures

pressure measured in both arms serves as a screen for subclavian stenosis; a systolic pressure difference of more than 10 mm Hg suggests significant subclavian disease. If subclavian artery stenosis is suspected and it is determined that the patient needs coronary bypass surgery, angiography is necessary to assess the suitability of using the left internal mammary artery as a bypass graft. Patients under consideration for a radial access approach should undergo an Allen's test (see Chapter 2). A focused physical examination also includes an assessment of the airway and documentation of the American Society of Anesthesiologists (ASA) Classification to determine the suitability for conscious sedation (Tables 1-2 and 1-3).

Several laboratory parameters routinely evaluated before cardiac catheterization include a complete blood count with platelets and levels of serum glucose, electrolytes, blood urea nitrogen, and creatinine. Patients who take warfarin and patients with liver disease, severe right-sided heart failure, or history of bleeding disorder require measurement of a prothrombin time usually expressed as an international normalized ratio (INR). All women of childbearing potential should have a serum pregnancy test checked before exposing them to radiation and potentially teratogenic medications. Laboratory values considered acceptable for catheterization are listed in Table 1-4; patients with laboratory values outside these parameters should not undergo elective catheterization until these abnormalities are addressed. In addition, the risk-benefit ratio of the procedure should be carefully considered for patients with other forms of laboratory derangement (e.g., marked hyperglycemia,

Table 1-2. **Airway Examination before Conscious Sedation**

1. Examine head and neck for abnormalities that lead to difficult intubation
   a. Neck range of motion (flexion and extension at least 35 degrees)
   b. Cervical spine instability or fusion
   c. Ability to open mouth
   d. Temporomandibular joint movement
   e. Mandible-hyoid bone distance (space between chin and notch of the thyroid cartilage with neck extended)
      • Adequate space is about 7 cm
      • Distance <7 cm is associated with more difficult intubation

2. Craniofacial abnormalities
   a. Congenital abnormalities
   b. Previous head or neck surgeries
   c. Previous head or neck radiation

3. Dentition and oral cavity
   a. Note missing, chipped, or loose teeth
   b. May need to remove partials for procedure
   c. Is uvula easily visualized when patient protrudes tongue?

Table 1-3.	American Society of Anesthesiologists Classification

Class I

Class I includes patients with no organic, physiologic, biochemical, or psychiatric disturbances. The pathologic process to be treated is localized and does not entail a systemic disease.

Class II

Class II includes patients with mild systemic disease caused by either the condition to be treated or by other pathophysiologic processes (i.e., irritable airway caused by tobacco abuse). No functional limitations.

Class III

Class III includes patients with severe systemic disease from any cause, even though it may not be possible to de fine the degree of disability with finality. Examples are limiting organic heart disease, diabetes with vascular com- plications, moderate-to-severe degrees of pulmonary insufficiency, and obesity that may limit airway and respira- tory management.

Class IV

Class IV includes patients with severe systemic disease not a constant threat to life. Examples include hospitalized patient with heart failure or persistent anginal syndrome and advanced degrees of pulmonary, hepatic, renal, or endocrine insufficiency.

Class V

Class V includes moribund patients not expected to survive without the operation/procedure. Conditions include profound shock, massive pulmonary embolism, ruptured blood vessels, and cerebral trauma with increasing intra- cranial pressure.

hyponatremia, acidosis). In general, for stable patients without a clinical suspicion of changing laboratory parameters (i.e., bleeding, renal failure, diuretic therapy), laboratory values no older than 30 days are acceptable.

Informed Consent. Informed consent is an extremely important part of the procedure and must be obtained for all patients before administration of conscious sedation. The physi- cian begins by describing the planned procedure in layman's terms with the patient and the family. Then, the physician discusses the risks of conscious sedation, catheterization, and coronary intervention in appropriate detail. Providing informed consent takes great commu- nication and interpersonal skills, and it is an important part of the procedure. Every patient deserves to hear the common potential complications of diagnostic cardiac catheterization (Table 1-5); these complications are discussed in greater detail in Chapter 3. The risks should not be glossed over or minimized. Patient dissatisfaction and potential lawsuits often arise from unexpected and improperly addressed minor complications. Depending on the patient's associated comorbidity, the likelihood of development of a serious complication might be higher than usual; the consent process should reflect this. For example, a patient with diabe- tes with a serum creatinine level of 3.0 mg/dL with multiple unmarked saphenous vein grafts should clearly understand the potential risk for development of further renal failure possibly

Table 1-4.	Common Laboratory Values Acceptable for Elective Cardiac Catheterization

LABORATORY TEST	VALUE
Prothrombin time (international normalized ratio)	<1.6 for routine catheterization procedures <1.2 if associated thrombocytopenia <1.1 if transseptal catheterization or myocardial biopsy
Potassium level	3.2–5.8 mmol/L
Serum creatinine level	<1.5 mg/dL
Hematocrit	>28%
Platelet count	>100,000/mm^3

Table 1-5.	Risks of Cardiac Catheterization	
COMPLICATION	FREQUENCY RANGE
Serious complications 　Death, myocardial infarction, 　stroke	0.1–0.4%
Vascular access site complication 　Bleeding 　Vessel Injury 　Hematoma 　Pseudoaneurysm 　Arterial thrombosis	1–6%
Renal failure	1–5%
Contrast allergy	0.1–0.5%
Risk of conscious sedation 　Respiratory failure	0.1–0.5%
Miscellaneous 　Infection 　Cardiac perforation 　Catheter entrapment 　Nerve injury 　Pulmonary embolism	Rare (<0.1%)

requiring dialysis after the procedure. Under no circumstance should a physician "talk a patient into" cardiac catheterization. Finally, a realistic and frank description of the risks involved is important, but it must be tailored to the patient. Some patients require a detailed and careful explanation of each potential risk; others need more in the way of reassurance when each risk is explained, sparing them graphic details.

Planning the Appropriate Procedure. Based on the precatheterization evaluation, the physician should determine the site of vascular access and plan the exact procedure to be performed. It should be determined whether a right heart catheterization is indicated. In general, any patient with a heart failure syndrome, unexplained dyspnea or edema, congenital heart disease, pericardial disease, or valvular heart disease, and any patient under evaluation for a heart, lung, or liver transplantation may require a right heart catheterization. Similarly, patients with unusual chest pain syndromes may need a right heart catheterization to exclude pulmonary hypertension. Patients undergoing catheterization primarily for the evaluation of recent acute myocardial infarction, stable or unstable angina, or chest pain syndromes without heart failure, hypotension, edema, or suspicion of a mechanical complication generally do not require right heart catheterization.

The location of vascular access should be decided. Most operators in the United States use the right or left femoral artery for arterial access. The presence of an arterial bruit in a patient with peripheral vascular disease does not exclude that artery as a site as long as a femoral pulse is present. In general, the presence of previous arterial bypass surgery (femoral-popliteal bypass or aortobifemoral bypass) does not exclude those locations as a possible access site but should be avoided if possible, particularly if surgery has been recent. Gaining central aortic access from the femoral region in the presence of a femoral-femoral or axillary-femoral bypass may prove difficult or impossible in some patients and should be avoided. Brachial artery access is reserved for patients with extensive vascular disease and no arterial pulses in the femoral region, and possibly patients who have had bilateral femoral vascular surgery. Radial artery access is becoming increasingly popular and can be considered in patients with peripheral vascular disease but may also be used routinely as an alternative to femoral access. Radial or brachial artery punctures are also performed for patients with morbid obesity or inability to lie flat for the procedure (e.g., in patients with severe lung disease or lower back conditions).

The type of contrast agent should be determined. A more detailed discussion regarding the different iodinated contrast agents is presented in Chapter 10. Most diagnostic catheterization laboratories use nonionic agents. The more expensive, nonionic, isosmolar contrast agents are used in patients with renal insufficiency or who undergo peripheral angiography because of less irritation. In patients with renal failure, use of a biplane laboratory, if available, may help reduce contrast use and decrease the likelihood of contrast-induced nephropathy.

It should be assumed that all patients who undergo left heart catheterization also undergo left ventriculography. Important exceptions include patients with renal failure in whom it is desirable to limit contrast volume, patients with decompensated heart failure and abnormal hemodynamics (i.e., left ventricular end diastolic pressure > 30 mm Hg) who may not tolerate the additional volume of contrast, and patients with severe aortic stenosis. Most patients who undergo left heart catheterization will undergo coronary angiography. Some rare circumstances include young patients without coronary risk factors referred for evaluation of congenital or valvular heart disease.

Aortography of the aortic root and thoracic aorta may be performed in patients with aortic regurgitation or a thoracic aortic aneurysm. Abdominal aortography is often performed as a screening test for suspected renal artery stenosis at the time of cardiac catheterization in patients with uncontrolled blood pressures refractory to multiple antihypertensive agents or in other situations in which renal artery stenosis is suspected. Selective renal angiography and intervention and abdominal aortography, and lower extremity runoff procedures for peripheral vascular disease are not usually combined with a diagnostic cardiac procedure except in special circumstances because of the concern about excessive contrast exposure and the risk of multiple procedures at one sitting.

Right ventricular biopsies are performed primarily in patients who have had cardiac transplantation. Endomyocardial biopsies in patients without transplantation carry a greater risk for perforation. These are occasionally performed during the diagnostic evaluation of patients with heart failure.

Patients with coronary disease who require bypass surgery found to have a subclavian bruit or a reduction in arterial blood pressure in the left arm relative to the right arm should undergo subclavian angiography to determine the presence of disease in the subclavian artery that might alter the use of the left internal mammary for bypass surgery. In addition, internal mammary angiography should be considered in patients who require repeat coronary bypass surgery or in patients who have had prior thoracotomy or chest wall irradiation to be sure there was no damage to the left internal mammary.

During diagnostic catheterization, trans-septal left heart catheterization is required in patients with a mechanical aortic prosthesis in whom it is necessary to measure left heart pressures (e.g., to assess transaortic or transmitral gradient) or to perform left ventriculography. Other diagnostic indications for trans-septal catheterization include the need to precisely determine left atrial pressure in a patient with suspected mitral stenosis or the desire to avoid crossing the aortic valve retrograde in patients with severe aortic stenosis. Trans-septal procedures are used extensively to perform many electrophysiologic procedures, mitral balloon valvuloplasty and new interventional procedures such as closure of atrial septal defect and patent foramen ovale, percutaneous mitral valve repair, insertion of a percutaneous left ventricular assist device, and delivery of left atrial appendage exclusion devices. Valve fluoroscopy is another procedure occasionally performed in the catheter laboratory to evaluate for mechanical valve thrombosis or malfunction.

Preprocedural Orders. Commonly used physician orders before routine cardiac catheterization are listed in Table 1-6. In addition to these, most physicians recommend holding all oral hypoglycemic agents and giving a half dose of long-acting (NPH) insulin on the morning of the procedure; patients with an insulin pump should be kept at the prescribed basal rate throughout the procedure and their procedure planned early in the day to avoid a prolonged fasting state. Because of the potential for dehydration, consider holding any

Table 1-6.	Preprocedural Orders

1. No solid food after midnight the night before the procedure

2. May have clear liquids until 0600 the morning of procedure and then nothing by mouth except for medications

3. If patient is to undergo an afternoon procedure, then a clear liquid breakfast is acceptable with nothing by mouth after that except for medications

4. Begin an intravenous infusion of 0.9% NaCl at 100 mL/hr

5. For patients at risk for contrast-induced nephropathy, initiate renal protection protocol (1)

6. For patients with history of contrast allergy: prednisone 60 mg by mouth the night before and the morning of the procedure; diphenhydramine 50 mg by mouth or intravenously just before the procedure

7. Consider an oral sedative just before the procedure (benzodiazepine)

8. Instruct the cardiac catheterization laboratory personnel to prepare the vascular access site

---

regularly scheduled diuretics. Intravenous heparin infusions are usually continued until just before the procedure. Similarly, for patients with acute coronary syndromes, the intravenous platelet glycoprotein IIb/IIIa inhibitors should not be interrupted. Warfarin is routinely held at least 48 to 72 hours before procedure with INR checks as noted earlier. For renal transplant patients taking cyclosporine or FK506 (Prograf), the morning dose before catheterization is typically held to minimize vasoconstriction and resumed the following day.

Postprocedural Orders. Postprocedure orders are important to help minimize potential complications. Commonly used orders are listed in Table 1-7. Management and monitoring of the vascular access site after the procedure is the most important aspect of these orders.

Table 1-7.	Postprocedural Orders

1. Intravenous fluids: 0.9 NaCl 1 L at 150 mL/hr to finish present bag, then convert to saline lock or at "keep vein open" rate until sheaths removed

2. Once sheath has been removed, encourage fluids by mouth

3. Temperature on return to unit

4. **Before arterial sheath removal:**
   a. Bed rest and nothing by mouth
   b. Check vital signs (blood pressure and heart rate) and the affected limb temperature and sensation, distal pulses, and cannulation site for hematoma or bleeding every 15 minutes for 1 hour, then every 30 minutes for 1 hour, then every 1 hour for 2 hours, then every 2 hours until sheaths removed
   c. If patient received heparin, sheath to be removed when activated clotting time <180 seconds

5. **After arterial sheath removal**
   a. For femoral approach: bed rest for 2–4 hours with affected limb straight after sheath removal and dressing applied; the head of bed may be raised 30–60 degrees and may logroll patient side to side, then increase activity as tolerated; at completion of bed rest, obtain orthostatic vital signs before ambulation
   b. For brachial/radial approach: bed rest with affected limb flexed at chest at 90 degrees until 2 hours after sheath removal and dressing applied; assess capillary refill and sensation in hand, radial pulse (in brachial access), ulnar pulse (in radial access), and cannulation site for hematoma or bleeding; head of bed may be raised 90 degrees and patient may turn side to side, then increase activity as tolerated; at completion of bed rest, obtain orthostatic vital signs before ambulation
   c. For patients with arterial closure device: bed rest for 1–2 hours after arterial sheath removal and dressing applied; head of bed may be raised 60 degrees; patient may freely move in bed immediately after procedure as long as there is no bleeding at access site; at completion of bedrest, obtain orthostatic vital signs before ambulation
   d. When sheaths removed, check vital signs, distal pulses, access site, cannulated limb temperature, and sensation every 15 minutes for 1 hour, then every 30 minutes for 1 hour, then every 1 hour for 2 hours

6. May place bladder catheter for inability to void while on bed rest; discontinue at completion of bedrest

7. At completion of bed rest, remove adhesive dressing (if any) and evaluate site for hematoma, bruit, ecchymosis, or rash

8. Call physician for any change in pulses or appearance of cannulated limb from baseline, bleeding from site, hematoma formation, hypotension, chills, fever, or chest pain suggestive of angina, change in extremity temperature, mottling, paresthesia or pain in affected extremity, or blood pressure <90 mm Hg

9. Medications: analgesics for procedural pain, antacids, medication for nausea, sleeping aids

10. Order diet

Often, trained nurses or technical personnel remove arterial sheaths. At some institutions, sheath removal by less experienced individuals in certain "high-risk" patients may not be appropriate. These include patients with severe aortic stenosis or severe aortic regurgitation, severe left main stenosis, coagulopathy or thrombocytopenia, presence of a large access site hematoma, severe hypertension, morbid obesity, or severe peripheral vascular disease.

At least one patient visit after the procedure is important to determine the presence of any periprocedural complications such as dye reactions, subtle neurologic complications, and vascular complications. This visit also provides the patient an opportunity to ask questions regarding his or her procedure. Activity is typically restricted for 2 days after cardiac catheterization.

Reference

1. Schweiger MJ, Chambers CE, Davidson CJ, et al: Prevention of contrast induced nephropathy: Recommendations for the high risk patient undergoing cardiovascular procedures. Catheter Cardiovasc Interv 2007;69:135–140.

CHAPTER 2

VASCULAR ACCESS AND HEMOSTASIS

All cardiac catheterization procedures begin with obtaining vascular access and end with achieving hemostasis. These two steps are often considered trivial, yet they arguably constitute the most important parts of the procedure. Vascular complications remain the most common cause of morbidity from cardiac catheterization, with several of them potentially life-threatening. Most complications are related to improper technique for gaining access or achieving hemostasis.

General Considerations in Obtaining Vascular Access. Choosing the arterial or venous access site is the first major decision facing a physician during cardiac catheterization. In the United States, the right femoral artery and vein are the most common access sites; the right internal jugular vein is the most common site when right heart catheterization alone is performed. The operator may seek alternatives to these sites depending on several important patient characteristics. For example, significant obesity may lead to difficulties with femoral access; radial access may be easier and reduce risk in such patients. The presence of peripheral vascular disease, prior vascular surgery, or intervention may prevent access via the usual route and require use of an alternative site. The risk for bleeding is another important variable. Patients at greater risk for bleeding (e.g., lytic state; severe, uncorrectable coagulopathy; marked thrombocytopenia) require careful planning regarding the access site. Finally, patient comfort is an important consideration, and an inability for a patient to lie flat may necessitate brachial or radial approaches instead of a femoral site.

Equipment Choices. A variety of needles, guide wires, and sheaths are available for securing arterial or venous access. The classic method of obtaining arterial access uses a two-piece, hollow-core needle with an obturator (Seldinger needle or modified Potts needle) to puncture the artery. This has mostly been abandoned by most operators for a one-piece, hollow-core needle without an obturator. Once an artery or vein has been successfully punctured, a guide wire is advanced through the lumen and the needle removed. Usually, a 0.035-inch, 145-cm-long J wire is used for the artery. Note that the standard J wire has a 3-mm diameter "J" loop. This may be too large when accessing smaller diameter arteries, necessitating the use of a smaller diameter J loop (1.5 mm). In the presence of peripheral vascular disease or vessel tortuosity, hydrophilic coated wires or "glide wires" are useful. Sheaths are used to secure access. Most cardiac catheterizations and interventions use 11-cm-long, 5- to 8-French (Fr) sheaths. Longer sheaths (24, 45, or 80 cm) are useful when there is iliac disease or severe vessel tortuosity, and larger diameter sheaths are available to perform some specific procedures. The sheath size refers to the internal lumen of the sheath (Table 2-1). The outer diameter of the sheath (i.e., the size of the hole it will make in the artery or vein) is larger than the stated French size of the sheath. In general, the external diameter of the sheath is 2 French sizes

Table 2-1.	Inner and Outer Diameters of Various Sheath Sizes	
SHEATH SIZE (FRENCH)	INNER DIAMETER	OUTER DIAMETER
5	1.7 mm/0.066 inch	7–8 French (Fr)
6	2.0 mm/0.079 inch	8–9 Fr
7	2.3 mm/0.092 inch	9–10 Fr
8	2.7 mm/0.105 inch	10–11 Fr
9	3.0 mm/0.118 inch	11–12 Fr
10	3.3 mm/0.131 inch	12–13 Fr

larger than the internal diameter of the sheath but may be larger or smaller depending on the specifications of the manufacturer. Many different sheaths are available on the market, with different properties useful to the operator such as hydrophilic coatings to ease passage and braided metal to prevent kinking.

Femoral Arterial Access. Left heart catheterization in the United States is most commonly performed from the femoral arteries. Nearly all vascular access is achieved using some form of the Seldinger technique, described in 1953 by the Swedish radiologist Sven-Ivar Seldinger (1921–1999). The essential steps of the Seldinger technique require puncture of the artery with a needle, passage of a guide wire through the needle lumen into the vessel, removal of the needle, and finally, replacement of the needle with a sheath or catheter.

To access the right femoral artery, the operator holds the needle with the right hand with the needle positioned between the thumb and index finger with a grip similar to holding a pencil. The index and middle fingers of the left hand are used to palpate the arterial pulse and anchor the artery. The needle is advanced at a 30- to 45-degree angle until arterial blood spurts in a pulsatile fashion from the end of the needle. The original technique used a needle with a solid obturator and intentionally passed the needle through the back wall of the artery, removing the obturator and slowly withdrawing until pulsatile blood returns. Most operators now try to puncture only the front wall of the artery. Blood should be freely pulsatile; if blood return is bright red but not pulsatile or only weakly pulsatile, the needle tip may be partially subintimal, against the wall or in a small side branch. Guide wire passage should not be attempted unless flow is brisk and pulsatile.

Once the operator is satisfied that the needle tip is within the lumen of the artery, the J-tipped guide wire is advanced through the needle lumen. The wire should pass freely with absolutely no resistance. The presence of resistance indicates a subintimal location of the needle tip, access of a small side branch instead of the appropriate vessel, or the presence of a stenosis. Difficulty passing a guide wire immediately on exiting the needle tip usually indicates a subintimal or side branch location and not a stenosis; the needle should be removed and arterial puncture reattempted. The wire should never be forced because this may result in subintimal passage and arterial dissection, vessel perforation, or plaque disruption.

With the guide wire in place in the distal aorta, the needle is withdrawn while gently applying pressure on the vessel with the left hand to prevent excess bleeding. The sheath is passed over the wire and inserted fully. Once the sheath is in place, the guide wire is removed. Again, there should be minimal or no resistance when passing the sheath over the guide wire. A small skin nick (2–3 mm) facilitates passage of the sheath. In the event of scarring from prior catheterization procedures, the operator may find that first passing a dilator alone can help allow a smoother sheath passage.

The target of the arterial puncture is the common femoral artery. Many major and potentially lethal vascular complications are related to punctures either above or below the common femoral artery. Retroperitoneal bleeds are almost entirely due to high punctures, whereas low punctures into either the profunda femoris or superficial femoral arteries are associated with hematoma, pseudoaneurysm, or arteriovenous fistula. Thus, it is imperative for the operator to understand the anatomy and major landmarks of the region when gaining access from the femoral location.

The normal anatomy of the femoral vessels and their relations to several important landmarks are shown in Figure 2-1. The inguinal ligament provides the boundary between the common femoral artery and the external iliac artery. The ideal puncture site is below the inguinal ligament and above the bifurcation of the common femoral artery into the profunda and superficial femoral arteries.

Identifying this specific site is not easy. External landmarks are completely unreliable. The commonly used technique of palpating the pubic symphysis and anterior iliac spine followed by mental visualization of the location of the inguinal ligament is inaccurate. Some operators puncture relative to the inguinal crease, made up of the skin fold between the abdomen and the groin. In the idealized (and nonexistent) patient with a normal body habitus, the inguinal crease lies 1 to 2 cm below the inguinal ligament. Based on this observation, puncture at or just below the inguinal crease is a commonly performed practice for accessing the femoral artery. However, the inguinal crease is entirely unreliable and should not form the basis of the puncture location. In obese patients, the inguinal crease may be many centimeters below the ligament, with puncture at the crease resulting in puncture of the profunda femoris or superficial femoral artery. In very thin patients, the crease may be higher than expected, causing puncture of the external iliac instead of the common femoral artery.

Bony landmarks, imaged fluoroscopically, form the most reliable landmarks to guide arterial puncture (1). The common femoral artery lies over the medial aspect of the femoral head (Fig. 2-2). Directing the puncture toward the center of the femoral head successfully accesses the common femoral artery in most cases (1). Fluoroscopic guidance must be done properly, however. It is not correct to fluoroscopically determine the relation between the femoral head and the position of a needle or hemostat simply placed on the surface of the skin. Because the needle enters at an angle and penetrates several centimeters of superficial tissue before entering the artery, arterial puncture occurs at a point several centimeters higher than the skin entry site. Therefore, if the puncture site is determined fluoroscopically by placing the needle on the skin surface, the actual site of the arterial puncture may occur above the inguinal ligament. This is particularly true for obese patients. It is more correct to pass a small-gauge "finder" needle to the level of the artery and then perform fluoroscopy to confirm the position (Fig. 2-3).

With the sheath in place, femoral arteriograms are helpful to determine the precise location of the puncture and are particularly useful when deciding on the method to achieve hemostasis, particularly in an anticoagulated patient. The ipsilateral oblique projection (20–30 degrees) is used most commonly (i.e., right anterior oblique for the right femoral artery and the left anterior oblique for punctures of the left femoral artery). The opposite oblique may be used if this view does not show the entry site or if branches overlap. The location of the inferior epigastric artery should be carefully noted on femoral angiography. This is a crucial landmark because puncture above the most inferior border of the inferior epigastric artery (not the site of origin of the branch) is associated with retroperitoneal bleed (Fig. 2-4) (2). Examples of femoral arteriograms showing both optimal punctures and punctures above and below the common femoral artery are shown in Videos 2-1, 2-2, and 2-3.

Special Considerations in Femoral Arterial Access. Several commonly encountered situations add complexity to femoral arterial access. These include the presence of iliac tortuosity, peripheral vascular disease, and coagulopathy.

Iliac tortuosity is commonly observed, particularly in elderly patients or patients with long-standing hypertension, and can create great difficulty with catheter manipulation. When obtaining access in such patients, the operator may encounter resistance during guide wire passage. In addition, it may be difficult to advance or to torque catheters, and efforts to do this may kink or knot the catheter. Use of a long sheath helps straighten the iliac vessels and facilitate catheter manipulation. An example of severe iliac tortuosity requiring a long sheath is shown in Figure 2-5.

Obtaining femoral arterial access in patients with peripheral vascular disease or prior vascular intervention or surgery may prove challenging. It is imperative to understand the precise nature of their disease or specifics of their prior vascular procedure before attempting arterial access. The presence of a bruit or established iliac or femoral stenosis does not necessarily exclude a site from consideration for access as long as the pulse is palpable. In general, the site with the strongest palpable pulse is chosen and care taken when advancing the guide wire. Fluoroscopic guidance ensures that the guide wire advances smoothly. If a J-tipped guide wire does not easily advance, a hydrophilic wire may prove successful. Hydrophilic wires used in conjunction with the access needle should proceed with great care because careless withdrawal of the wire through the needle may cut or damage the wire. In general, in the presence of prior vascular surgery or intervention, an alternative access site should be chosen. If unavoidable, the femoral approach is acceptable more than 3 months after placement of iliac stents, or aortic stent grafts, or after aortofemoral, or aortoiliac bypass surgery. In the presence of femoral-femoral bypass or femoral-popliteal bypass, it is probably best to use the brachial or radial approach.

Patients with coagulopathy or platelet disorders are at an increased risk for access site bleeding and access-related complications. If possible, these disturbances should be corrected before catheterization. This is not always possible either because the procedure is emergent or because the coagulopathy cannot be readily corrected (e.g., in patients with hepatic cirrhosis). For elective procedures, the cutoff values used at the University of Virginia include an international normalized ratio (INR) less than 1.6 and platelet count greater than 60,000/mm^3. When catheterization is necessary in a patient with coagulopathy or platelet disorder, several techniques can be used to reduce vascular complications. Fresh frozen plasma or platelet transfusion at the time of access and/or sheath removal may be necessary. Vascular closure devices may prove useful. In addition, the radial artery can be considered as an alternative access site. Prolonged bed rest after sheath removal may prevent bleeding complications.

Brachial Artery Access. The brachial artery provides an alternative to the femoral artery for left heart catheterization access (the left brachial artery is often chosen over the right brachial artery because the preformed coronary catheters engage easier). The brachial approach is chosen when femoral access is undesired, usually because of peripheral arterial disease. This route may also be preferred for morbidly obese patients, in patients unable to lie flat, or when a left internal mammary artery bypass graft cannot be selectively engaged from the femoral route.

Accessing the brachial artery is similar to the technique described for the femoral artery with a few important differences. Because the brachial artery is smaller in diameter, the puncture requires greater care. The surrounding tissue does not anchor the artery as securely, causing the brachial artery to "roll away" as the needle approaches. In addition, the J loop of the guide wire may exceed the inner diameter of the brachial artery creating difficult passage; a smaller diameter J wire or hydrophilic wire may be helpful in these cases. After insertion of the sheath, heparin is administered and the sheath frequently flushed to prevent thrombosis. Careful monitoring of the distal pulse should be performed during and after the procedure.

The brachial approach has a greater complication rate than the femoral approach. This is predominantly due to the fact that the brachial artery is smaller and an end-organ artery. Thrombosis of the brachial artery is more common than in the femoral artery and leads to acute, limb-threatening ischemia. Hematoma formation, usually well tolerated in the femoral area, may lead to compartment syndrome and limb ischemia. Median nerve injury is another unique complication of brachial access and is due to the close proximity of the nerve to the artery. Because of the greater complication rate associated with brachial artery catheterization, radial artery access is the preferred alternative to the femoral artery.

Radial Artery Access. In selected patients, the radial artery can be used as an alternative to femoral or brachial access. Catheterization from the radial artery may be technically more demanding for the operator and is associated with longer procedure times than the femoral approach; however, the vascular complication rate (particularly bleeding risk) is lower, and this site is associated with greater patient comfort because of less bed rest and shorter time lying flat than the traditional femoral artery approach.

The technique is not appropriate for all patients. The ulnar and radial arteries join to form the palmar arch, supplying the circulation to the hand. Before attempting radial access, the operator must first demonstrate that the ulnar artery is capable of supporting the circulation of the entire palmar arch (in the event of radial artery occlusion) by first performing the modified Allen's test. To perform this assessment, the examiner simultaneously compresses both the ulnar and radial arteries between thumb and index fingers while instructing the patient to repeatedly clench and open his or her fist until the hand blanches. The examiner then releases compression on the ulnar artery and determines the time it takes to restore the pink color of the hand; a normal response is within 10 seconds. Radial artery access is usually avoided if the Allen's test exceeds 10 seconds.

The radial approach is favored by some operators as the primary access site for cardiac catheterization, particularly outside the United States. Radial access is often used in morbidly obese patients and in patients with peripheral vascular disease or those who are unable to lie flat. In some patient groups, the radial approach may prove difficult. These groups include patients with prior bypass grafts, severe iliac tortuosity (because the subclavian arteries are often also affected), and patients who require large-caliber (>6 French) sheaths. The safety and success of repeat radial procedures is not well defined. Finally, because of the small (<5%) but definite chance of radial artery occlusion, this site should be avoided in patients in whom a radial artery is considered for a graft conduit.

Achieving radial artery access requires meticulous technique and modification of the method described for the femoral approach. After administering a small amount of local anesthesia over the radial artery, the operator uses a small needle (21 gauge) to puncture the artery. When arterial blood returns, a 0.018-inch guide wire is advanced under fluoroscopic guidance. The wire should pass easily to the brachial artery before advancing the sheath. Hydrophilic-coated sheaths are easier to position and remove than conventional sheaths. Many operators locally administer a combination of drugs to prevent or reverse spasm provoked by instrumentation. The University of Virginia laboratory uses a cocktail of 1 mg verapamil combined with 100 mcg nitroglycerine in 10 mL heparinized saline. The entire 10 mL is administered as a bolus through the arterial sheath, and up to 10 doses may be used during a case. Others have used a mixture of 5 mg verapamil and 200 mcg nitroglycerine or administer topical nitrates over the site. Once the sheath is placed, coronary catheters can be directed under fluoroscopic guidance into the ascending aorta with a 0.035-inch hydrophilic wire. From the radial approach, the end of the guide wire may preferentially enter the descending aorta. This often frustrating problem may be corrected by instructing the patient to take a deep breath allowing the wire and catheter to more easily enter the ascending aorta. Selective cannulation of the coronary arteries can be challenging, particularly for operators with more experience from the femoral approach. A different set of catheters is often required, especially for the left coronary artery. With experience, however, the radial approach can be readily mastered and provides a valuable alternative to the traditional femoral access site.

Complications of radial artery access are uncommon. The most frequent adverse event is forearm pain from radial artery spasm. In 5% to 10% of cases, the catheterization cannot be completed and the case converted to a femoral approach. Failure from the radial approach is often due to the presence of a radioulnar (also called *recurrent radial*) loop (Fig. 2-6). In the presence of a radioulnar loop, it may be difficult or impossible to safely pass a guide wire around the loop into the brachial or subclavian artery. Aggressive attempts at wire positioning may lead to vessel perforation or dissection, and in the event a guide wire is successfully positioned, catheter advancement and manipulation will likely prove impossible. Loops may be present at several locations in the radial artery. More rarely, they involve the brachial or subclavian arteries.

In addition to radioulnar loops, other anatomic variations or abnormalities that lead to inability to complete a catheterization from the radial approach include radial artery hypoplasia and subclavian or axillary tortuosity. The radial and ulnar arteries may branch high from the brachial artery, creating difficulty in passing catheters through the longer than usual and small-diameter radial artery. This may lead to complications such as dissection and inability to complete the case from the radial artery; an example of this is shown in Video 2-4. In some patients, it is not possible to successfully engage one or more of the coronary arteries; this problem substantially decreases with operator experience. Occlusion of the radial artery may occur in 2% to 5% of cases, and in the presence of an acceptable Allen's test, rarely results in symptoms. Rare complications include perforation of the radial artery or one of the small branches of the radial artery, hematoma, and possible compartment syndrome, and entrapment of the sheath or catheter caused by intense spasm. Case reports of avulsion of the radial artery and chronic regional pain syndrome have been reported.

Venous Access. Venous access is required to perform a right heart catheterization. The technique for achieving venous access is similar to that used for an artery with the exception that the venous pulse cannot be felt. The operator must rely on anatomic landmarks or adjacent arterial pulsations to guide the puncture. A hollow-core needle attached to a syringe is used to puncture the vein. When brisk venous return is confirmed, the J wire is advanced, the needle removed, and a sheath inserted over the guide wire.

The femoral vein is often used, particularly when a left heart catheterization from the femoral artery is also planned. The femoral vein arises behind the superficial femoral artery running medial to the common femoral artery (see Fig. 2-1). The operator easily achieves femoral venous access by first palpating the femoral arterial pulse and puncturing medial to it. The optimal entry site is the level of the common femoral artery. Punctures lower than this may inadvertently enter the artery, creating an arteriovenous fistula. The presence of an inferior vena caval filter placed to prevent pulmonary embolism in a patient with thromboembolic disease precludes the use of the femoral venous site for heart catheterization.

The internal jugular vein is an important access site for performing right heart catheterization. Typically, the right internal jugular vein is used. The associated anatomy of the internal jugular vein is shown in Figure 2-7. Several techniques have been proposed for accessing the internal jugular vein; one method is described as follows. With the patient in the supine position, the head is turned to the left. Placing the patient in the Trendelenburg position helps maximally engorge the vein and prevent air embolism if filling pressures are low. Important landmarks include the clavicle, the carotid artery, and the two heads of the sternocleidomastoid muscle (sternal and clavicular heads). The internal jugular vein runs in the triangle created by these two muscle heads. A 21-gauge needle attached to a syringe may be used as a "finder" needle. Although the optimal site in any given patient may vary, in general, the needle usually successfully enters the vein at the apex of the triangle created by the sternocleidomastoid about 2 cm above the clavicle, lateral to the sternal head. The needle should be directed toward the ipsilateral nipple at between 45 and 90 degrees to the neck. When the vein is entered with this finder needle, it is removed from the site. Repuncture is performed in the same manner using the larger bore, hollow-core needle, and a J-tipped guide wire is advanced when brisk venous blood is returned. The guide wire should pass easily with no resistance. The tip of the guide wire may enter the right ventricle necessitating monitoring for ventricular ectopy. A sheath is then placed over the guide wire as described earlier. If difficulty with access is encountered, ultrasound guidance is helpful at locating the vein (Fig. 2-8). Complications of internal jugular venous access include hematoma, carotid artery puncture, pneumothorax, brachial plexus injury, and hemothorax.

The brachial veins can also be used for right heart catheterization. In fact, this was the access site chosen for the first successful right heart catheterization performed by Dr. Werner Forssmann on himself in 1932. The brachial veins are particularly useful in patients already undergoing left heart catheterization from the arm (radial or brachial arterial access) or in patients with coagulopathy. It is important to use the medial veins because these communicate directly with the axillary and then subclavian venous system (Fig. 2-9). The lateral veins enter the axillary veins at angles that often preclude successful passage of a catheter to the heart.

Hemostasis. The ability to achieve hemostasis without complication depends on the quality of the initial puncture. Failure to achieve a front wall puncture is associated with bleeding from the arteriotomy in the posterior aspect of the vessel. Punctures above the inguinal ligament or below the bifurcation often cannot be easily compressed because the arteriotomy lies above or below the femoral head. Similarly, if initial access attempts resulted in arterial punctures but were not successful at achieving access or if there was inadvertent puncture of the vein, hemostasis of the ultimately successful arteriotomy site might be associated with ongoing bleeding from these other punctures, particularly in an anticoagulated patient. Thus, meticulous attention to achieving the highest quality arteriotomy will lead to the best vascular outcomes.

Manual compression remains the mainstay of hemostasis. The technique is fairly simple. With the sheath still in place, the arterial pulse is palpated above the sheath insertion site using the middle and index fingers of the left hand. The sheath is slowly removed with compression applied above the site using the left hand. Once the sheath is out, the index and middle fingers of the right hand are also used to compress the artery just below the puncture site. Compression should be applied with enough force to prevent bleeding; initially, this usually obliterates the distal pulse. Pressure should be slowly relieved to allow the palpation of the distal pulse yet still maintain hemostasis. Usually, 10 to 20 minutes of compression is required to achieve hemostasis in an unanticoagulated patient with a 6 to 8 Fr sheath. In patients who have received anticoagulation with heparin, an activated coagulation time of less than 180 seconds is required before manual compression performed. Prolonged manual compression is often needed in patients with larger caliber sheaths, excessive anticoagulation, arterial hypertension, severe aortic regurgitation, renal failure, thrombocytopenia, or platelet dysfunction. After successful manual compression, a period of bed rest is indicated until the arterial plug is stable. Usually 2 to 4 hours of bed rest is prescribed; ambulation may be initiated as early as 1 hour after successful hemostasis after catheterization with 5 Fr catheters in unanticoagulated patients (3).

Manual compression is an effective and inexpensive method for achieving hemostasis but requires human resources and is associated with greater patient discomfort, immobility, and time in bed. Vascular closure devices were first developed during the 1990s in an attempt to limit the bleeding associated with the institution of powerful adjunctive pharmacologic agents for percutaneous coronary intervention and to reduce patient immobility after catheterization procedures.

Numerous devices have been developed and are summarized in Table 2-2. Each technique has been shown to be effective at achieving hemostasis, and they appear to consistently

Table 2-2.	**Vascular Closure Devices**
Suture mediated	
Perclose (Abbott Vascular)	
Extravascular collagen	
Angio-Seal (St. Jude Medical)	
Staple mediated	
StarClose (Abbott Vascular)	
EVS-Angiolink (Medtronic)	
Passive or assisted closure	
Syvek Patch (Marine Polymer Technologies)	
FemoStop (Radi Medical)	

reduce time in bed and improve patient comfort compared with manual compression. Little randomized, controlled data comparing the efficacy and safety of the various vascular closure devices currently in use have been reported, and it is unclear whether these devices reduce vascular complication rates compared with manual compression (4, 5).

Vascular closure devices cannot be used in all patients. Many of the devices require confirmation by femoral angiography that the arteriotomy is in the common femoral artery, and many require a minimal femoral artery diameter of 4 mm. These devices should be used with great care in anticoagulated patients because failure of the device to achieve hemostasis will require prolonged manual compression and may be associated with increased risk for bleeding. For this reason, they should probably be avoided in patients with an arteriotomy above the inguinal ligament because failure of the device may be associated with retroperitoneal bleed. The suture-mediated closure devices are occasionally complicated by infection, a serious problem not observed in patients undergoing manual compression. Continued evolution and improvement of these devices is anticipated; their ultimate role in achieving hemostasis after routine catheterization and percutaneous intervention remains a subject of debate and study.

References

1. Schnyder G, Sawhney N, Whisenant B, et al: Common femoral artery anatomy is influenced by demographics and comorbidity: Implications for cardiac and peripheral invasive studies. Catheter Cardiovasc Interv 2001;53:289–295.
2. Sherev DA, Shaw RE, Brent BN: Angiographic predictors of femoral access site complications: Implications for planned percutaneous coronary intervention. Catheter Cardiovasc Interv 2005;65:196–202.
3. Doyle BJ, Konz BA, Lennon RJ, et al: Ambulation 1 hour after diagnostic cardiac catheterization: A prospective study of 1009 procedures. Mayo Clin Proc 2006;81:1537–1540.
4. Nikolsky E, Mehran R, Halkin A, et al: Vascular complications associated with arteriotomy closure devices in patients undergoing percutaneous coronary procedures. A meta-analysis. J Am Coll Cardiol 2004;44:1200–1209.
5. Dauerman HL, Applegate RJ, Cohen DJ: Vascular closure devices. The second decade. J Am Coll Cardiol 2007;50: 1617–1626.

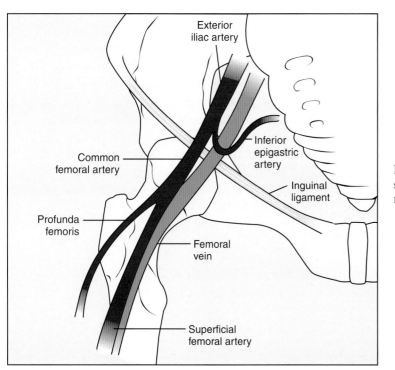

FIGURE 2-1. Normal anatomy of the femoral vessels and their relation to associated bony and ligamentous structures.

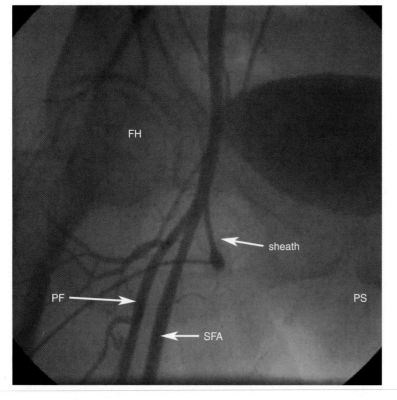

FIGURE 2-2. Right femoral angiogram performed through a femoral artery sheath demonstrating the important bony landmarks. The center of the femoral head (*FH*) is generally the optimal target for puncture of the common femoral artery (*CFA*) at a location below the inguinal ligament and above the bifurcation of the profunda femoris (*PF*) and superficial femoral artery (*SFA*). The pubic symphysis (*PS*) is the origin of the inguinal ligament.

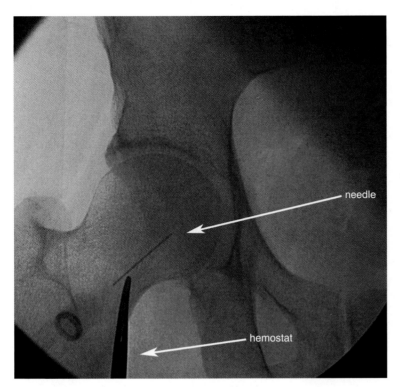

FIGURE 2-3. Relation between the skin entry site and arterial entry site on fluoroscopy. A hemostat is placed on the surface of the skin at the site where the needle enters the skin. The needle tip has entered the common femoral artery. Thus, when fluoroscopy is used to guide femoral artery puncture, the needle should be at the level of the artery and not simply be placed on the skin surface, because this may cause arterial puncture higher than intended.

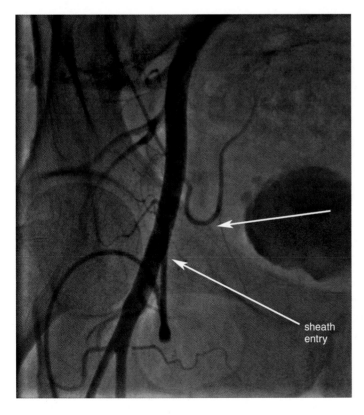

FIGURE 2-4. The inferior epigastric artery is an important landmark in femoral artery access. Puncture above the lower extent of the inferior epigastric artery *(arrow)* is associated with a greater risk for retroperitoneal bleed.

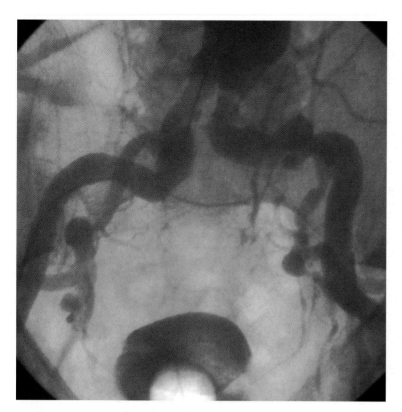

FIGURE 2-5. Angiogram displays an example of the marked iliac tortuosity that may be encountered during femoral artery access.

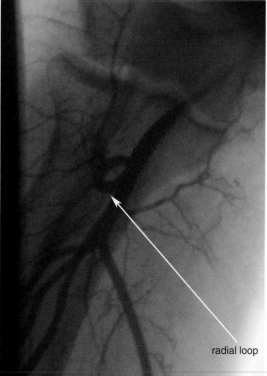

radial loop

FIGURE 2-6. Radial artery angiogram shows a recurrent radial loop (*arrow*). This finding generally precludes the use of the radial artery for cardiac catheterization.

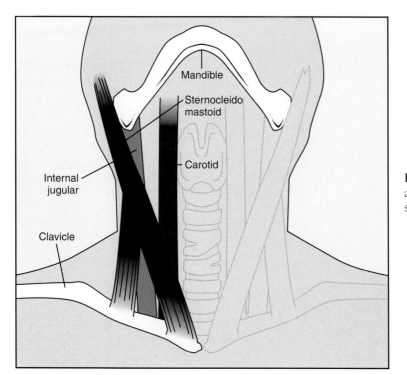

FIGURE 2-7. Normal anatomy of the jugular vein and its relation to associated vascular and muscular structures.

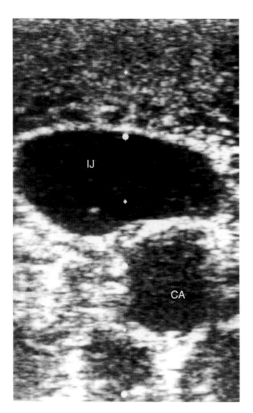

FIGURE 2-8. Ultrasound may prove helpful in accessing the internal jugular vein. The vein (*IJ*) is generally larger, more lateral, and more subject to respiratory changes than the carotid artery (*CA*).

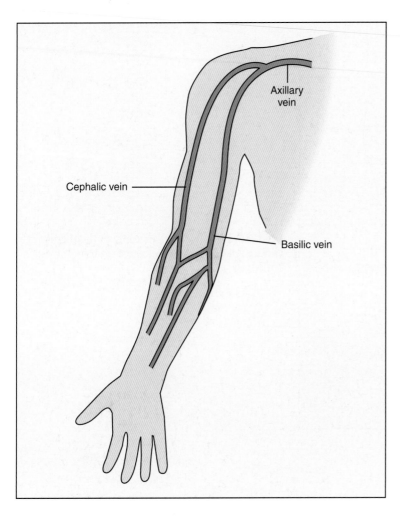

FIGURE 2-9. Normal anatomy of the brachial veins. Right heart catheterization may be successfully performed from the basilic vein, on the ulnar side of the forearm, but not the cephalic veins.

CHAPTER 3

COMPLICATIONS OF CARDIAC CATHETERIZATION

With more than 50 years of refinement and progress, diagnostic cardiac catheterization has become a safe procedure with a low complication rate. However, numerous potential life- and limb-threatening complications are associated with cardiac catheterization (Table 3-1). Fundamental to competency in performance of these procedures is an understanding of the causes and risk factors for complications, and knowledge of their recognition and treatment.

Incidence of Complications. The incidence of individual complications depends on the definition and methodology used to identify the complication (1). For example, unless cardiac isoenzymes are measured routinely, the incidence of a non–Q-wave myocardial infarction will be underestimated. Similarly, a significant hematoma can be variably defined based on size (e.g., >10 cm), a transfusion requirement, or as an event prolonging length of stay. Some serious consequences of a complication may not develop in the catheterization laboratory and may not be attributed to the procedure. These include some neurologic complications such as visual field defects often unrecognized until after the procedure or cholesterol embolization syndrome that may not be apparent until days after the procedure. The actual incidence of individual complications is further obscured by the methodology used to collect them. Published registries that rely on self-reporting of complications likely underestimate the true incidence of complications compared with more carefully performed studies using prospectively defined data collection. Nevertheless, after taking these important points into consideration, the approximate incidence of major complications is summarized in Table 3-2.

Of course, not all patients have the same likelihood of acquiring a complication. Patients with Class IV heart disease, poor left ventricular function, advanced age, left main coronary disease, or severe aortic stenosis are clearly at increased risk for a catheterization-related complication. Similarly, certain comorbid illnesses increase risk. Particularly important among these include end-stage renal failure, severe peripheral vascular disease, renal insufficiency, significant liver or pulmonary disease, and marked hematologic abnormalities such as thrombocytopenia or coagulopathy. In these patients, the risk-benefit ratio of cardiac catheterization should be carefully weighed before proceeding.

Mechanisms of Complications. Complications arise from one of several mechanisms: (a) complications from vascular access and hemostasis; (b) catheter-related injury to the coronary arteries, femoral or iliac vessels, or aorta; (c) embolization of thrombus, air, or atheromatous debris; (d) toxicity from drugs used in the catheterization laboratory or from radiocontrast agents; and (e) exacerbation or unmasking of underlying conditions from the catheterization procedure. Examples of the latter include hemodynamic deterioration after

Table 3-1. Selected Potential Complications of Cardiac Catheterization

Death

Cerebrovascular accident

Myocardial infarction

Emergency bypass surgery

Respiratory compromise
Pulmonary edema
Oversedation

Hypotension

Arrhythmia

Vascular or access-related complications
    Bleeding
    Retroperitoneal bleeding
    Hematoma
    Pseudoaneurysm
    Arteriovenous fistula
    Arterial thrombosis
    Vessel injury (dissection, perforation)
    Compartment syndrome
    Nerve injury

Allergic reaction

Renal failure

Miscellaneous and unusual complications
    Deep venous thrombosis/pulmonary embolism
    Infection
    Chamber of vessel perforation
    Catheter entrapment
    Cholesterol embolization
    Radiation-induced skin injury
    Air embolism

ventriculography in patients with severe aortic stenosis, induction of ischemia after coronary angiography in patients with critical underlying coronary artery disease, and precipitation of pulmonary edema in patients with poor ventricular function.

Review of Specific Complications: Death. Procedural death (i.e., during cardiac catheterization) rarely occurs (<1/1000). When death occurs in the cardiac catheterization laboratory, it is usually a consequence of a catastrophic event such as pulmonary artery rupture, massive air embolism, cardiac perforation, catheter-related dissection of a coronary artery, or disruption of a left main stem plaque. These events are fortunately rare and usually preventable with careful attention to detail and meticulous technique. Other potential mechanisms

Table 3-2. Incidence of Common Complications of Cardiac Catheterization

COMPLICATION	INCIDENCE
Death	0.1–0.2%
Myocardial infarction	0.1%
Cerebrovascular accident	<0.4%
Vascular complication	2–5%
Severe contrast reaction	<0.2%
Minor contrast reaction	3–12%
Renal failure	1–30%

include anaphylaxis from contrast or development of refractory arrhythmias. Some deaths occur either as a consequence of the natural history of the illness for which they are undergoing catheterization (e.g., cardiogenic shock) or from a catheterization-provoked exacerbation of the underlying cardiac condition. The latter scenario is particularly relevant to patients with severe aortic stenosis in whom even a slight perturbation caused by the catheterization procedure, such as hypotension from procedural-induced dehydration, sedation, or contrast-induced vasodilatation, may trigger a cascade of detrimental events leading to their demise.

Catheter-induced injury of the left main coronary artery is usually due to dissection and can occur when the catheter used to engage the left main coronary ostium is of an incorrect size or if it lunges into the artery with too great a force. Dissection may rapidly lead to closure of the artery. A similar event may occur when a catheter engages the artery and inadvertently disrupts a plaque located in the left main ostium, causing acute closure of the artery. In both cases, left main occlusion rapidly leads to profound ischemia, hemodynamic collapse, and death unless promptly treated. Video 3-1 shows an example of a patient who experienced development of abrupt closure of the left main artery after a diagnostic catheter engaged the vessel and angiography demonstrated severe ostial disease of the left main stem causing immediate cardiovascular collapse. The artery was stented quickly, and the patient fortunately survived.

Cerebrovascular Accident. Stroke is a rare but dreaded complication of cardiac catheterization. Depending on the definition used, the reported incidence rate varies from 0.05% to 0.4% (2). Most strokes from catheterization represent an embolic event from atheromatous debris inadvertently loosened from the aorta during passage of catheters. A stroke may also occur if debris or thrombus from the aortic valve or left ventricular cavity is disrupted during the process of catheterization. These events are mostly unavoidable and represent an unfortunate but intrinsic risk of the procedure. Improper technique may contribute to some events. Thrombus or air introduced by the catheter may embolize causing a stroke. Intracranial bleed is only rarely responsible for an acute neurologic event from catheterization but should be considered in patients receiving anticoagulant therapy at the time of a catheterization or intervention.

It is difficult to identify patients likely to have a stroke from catheterization before the procedure. The presence of extensive aortic disease is a well-known risk factor and may be apparent on fluoroscopy (Fig. 3-1). This finding, also known as a *porcelain aorta,* is predictive of stroke and embolism during bypass surgery.

Myocardial Infarction. Myocardial infarction is a rarely reported complication of diagnostic catheterization but is likely under-represented because serologic markers of myonecrosis are not routinely measured after catheterization. Several mechanisms account for this complication, including catheter injury, embolization of clot, air or atheromatous debris, and precipitation of severe ischemia from catheter placement or contrast injection in the presence of severe, underlying coronary disease.

The current generation of diagnostic catheters is safe and rarely results in catheter-related injury. However, catheters can traumatize the intima of a coronary artery causing dissection and potentially leading to ischemia and infarction from transient closure of the vessel. As noted earlier, if the left main artery is involved, this complication may be catastrophic and have a fatal outcome. Most catheter-related dissections are related to improper catheter positioning; thus, it is important to achieve coaxial alignment of the catheter. In the case of the left coronary artery, if the Judkins catheter is too short, the tip will be positioned at a sharp angle toward the superior aspect of the left main artery possibly disrupting the intima (Video 3-2). Furthermore, a forceful contrast injection in such a position can extend the dissection, worsening the problem. Catheter engagement of the right coronary artery, particularly when the left Amplatz catheter is used, may cause dissection and closure because efforts to engage the artery may cause the catheter to rapidly lunge down the coronary artery disrupting the intima.

Embolization of debris, air, or thrombus is a more common mechanism for procedural-related infarction. Most of these are due to inattention or improper technique. During cardiac catheterization, thrombus may form on guide wires and within the arterial sheaths or diagnostic catheters. Careful aspiration and flushing of catheters is important to prevent this, particularly when a guide wire has been used. The inability to aspirate a catheter after removing the guide wire and observing damping of the pressure waveform are important clues to the presence of a clot within the catheter. If unsuspected, they may embolize down a coronary artery during injection and lead to an acute infarction.

Respiratory Failure. Respiratory failure during catheterization may be caused by oversedation, anaphylaxis to contrast, acute pulmonary edema, or exacerbation of underlying lung or heart disease. This complication can be minimized by careful assessment of the patient before catheterization, avoiding large contrast volumes in patients with abnormal hemodynamics or poor left ventricular function, and careful monitoring of the patient's respiratory status after administration of sedatives.

Arrhythmia. Arrhythmias are common during catheterization; most are benign and without clinical sequelae. A full spectrum of arrhythmias may occur including ventricular fibrillation, ventricular tachycardia, atrial arrhythmias, heart block, bradyarrhythmia, and asystole. Arrhythmias often result from contrast toxicity and were more commonly observed with the older ionic than with the newer nonionic or isosmolar agents. Arrhythmias may also occur as a consequence of poor injection technique or from the unmasking of ischemia in the presence of underlying coronary disease. Improper catheter position or overinjection of contrast during coronary angiography is a common cause of transient arrhythmia including ventricular fibrillation. This complication is typically observed when contrast is carelessly injected into the conus branch of the right coronary artery or into a nondominant right coronary artery (Video 3-3). Another frequent cause of arrhythmia during catheterization is from catheter position in cardiac chambers. Complete heart block may occur while crossing an aortic valve, particularly if there is an underlying right bundle branch block. Similarly, complete heart block may develop when a Swan–Ganz catheter is passed through the right ventricle into the pulmonary outflow tract in patients with an underlying left bundle branch block. Atrial and ventricular arrhythmias are often seen when catheters are placed in the cardiac chambers; most of the time, rhythm disturbances are transient and self-limited, but occasionally the catheters trigger a sustained arrhythmia requiring correction. For this reason, cardiac catheterization is always performed under electrocardiographic monitoring.

Hypotension. Familiarity with the broad differential diagnosis of hypotension after catheterization is important (Table 3-3). Some of the causes, such as hypovolemia and dehydration, are benign and easily correctable, whereas others, such as retroperitoneal bleed or anaphylaxis, are potentially life-threatening. After assessing the patient, it is reasonable to first consider a fluid bolus. If the blood pressure is not quickly restored, the physician should carefully consider the other, more serious causes.

Vascular Complications. Vascular complications remain one of the most common sources of morbidity, patient dissatisfaction, and medicolegal liability from catheterization. Risk factors include the use of anticoagulants, the presence of platelet dysfunction or coagulopathy, and the presence of underlying vascular disease. Perhaps the most important determinant of vascular complications relates to the use of improper technique for obtaining access or for achieving hemostasis.

Retroperitoneal bleeding is a rare (<0.5% of catheterizations) but serious and life-threatening vascular complication of femoral artery catheterization (3, 4). It is typically caused by inadvertent arterial puncture above the inguinal ligament (Fig. 3-2). The problem usually becomes manifest when the arterial sheath is removed. A puncture at this location is difficult or impossible to compress because there is no bony structure (i.e., the femoral head) to provide support for the compression. The problem is further compounded by the fact that continued bleeding is not recognized by the operator because the blood enters the retroperitoneal space giving the false impression that hemostasis has been achieved. The bleeding is not usually identified until there are hemodynamic sequelae. Retroperitoneal bleeding also arises

Table 3-3. **Causes of Hypotension Complicating Cardiac Catheterization**

Drug related (sedatives, nitrates, among others)

Anaphylaxis from contrast

Dehydration

Vasovagal reaction

Bleeding
   Retroperitoneal bleed
   Hematoma
   Occult gastrointestinal bleed

Cardiac tamponade from unrecognized perforation

Ischemia from iatrogenic injury to left main or right coronary artery

Cardiogenic shock

Arrhythmia

Other
   Air embolism
   Cerebrovascular accident
   Aortic dissection
   Pulmonary embolism

from laceration of the small branches around the common femoral artery, puncture of the inferior epigastric artery, or perforation of the iliac artery during sheath or catheter manipulation during the procedure. Bleeding may also arise spontaneously from anticoagulation used during coronary intervention.

The diagnosis is readily made on clinical grounds. It classically manifests as unexplained hypotension or vagal reaction either during the procedure or shortly after the arterial sheath is removed. Back, flank, or suprainguinal pain and a decline in hematocrit are common. Compression of the femoral nerve from the expanding retroperitoneal hematoma may cause a neuropathy. Adjunctive imaging with computerized tomographic scanning can be used to confirm the clinical diagnosis but is not necessary in most cases. It should be noted that patients clinically suspected to have retroperitoneal bleeding who are hemodynamically unstable should probably not undergo computed tomographic scanning until they are stabilized. Retroperitoneal bleeding is successfully managed in most cases by aggressive volume resuscitation, correction of coagulopathy, and transfusion of packed red blood cells to maintain the hematocrit. Vascular surgery consult obtained early on is helpful, although surgery is only rarely necessary (16% of cases in one series) and is reserved for hypotension unresponsive to volume or progressive decline in hematocrit despite transfusion (3). As an alternative to surgery, a covered stent may be placed from the opposite femoral artery to seal the puncture site and control the bleeding.

Hematomas are the most common vascular complication and are due to bleeding from the puncture site often occurring when vascular sheaths are removed. Many are small with little or no clinical consequence. Large hematomas (e.g., >8cm) may cause a significant decline in hematocrit, hypotension, and discomfort. Large hematomas may lead to other, potentially serious problems such as compartment syndrome, nerve compression, deep venous thrombosis, and cellulitis. In addition, a hematoma may be associated with a pseudoaneurysm, further complicating the course.

Many groin hematomas are caused by puncture below the common femoral artery into either the profunda femoris or superficial femoral artery branches. Hematomas can be minimized by taking steps to ensure entry into the common femoral artery and by adopting meticulous technique at obtaining hemostasis. Avoiding or minimizing the use of postprocedural anticoagulation also helps prevent this complication. Treatment is generally conservative and supportive; large, expanding hematomas, or ones associated with compartment syndrome or nerve compression may require surgical evacuation.

Pseudoaneurysms complicate about 0.5% of catheterization procedures and arise when there is bleeding at the arterial access entry site and the creation of a hematoma with flow from the artery passing through the arteriotomy site into the hematoma. The lesion is called a *pseudoaneurysm* because the wall of the aneurysm consists solely of fibrin and not arterial vessel. Pseudoaneurysms typically form when the puncture site is below the common femoral artery, if hemostasis has been improperly performed, or if anticoagulation is resumed after sheath removal. The diagnosis is often made clinically when a painful, pulsatile mass over the access site and a systolic bruit are noted. Ultrasound is necessary to confirm the diagnosis, define the size of the pseudoaneurysm, and guide its management. An example of a pseudoaneurysm detected during femoral angiography is shown in Video 3-4.

Adverse consequences of a pseudoaneurysm include rebleeding and rupture with massive hemorrhage, extension of a hematoma, infection, and development of a compressive neuropathy. Small femoral pseudoaneurysms (<1 cm) may close spontaneously with bed rest. Traditionally, femoral artery pseudoaneurysms have been repaired by vascular surgeons. This has been replaced by the use of thrombin injection directly into the pseudoaneurysm chamber with surgery reserved for cases that cannot be treated or fail to close by this method (5).

Arteriovenous fistulae complicate up to 0.9% of cardiac catheterizations (6). This complication often originates from a puncture below the common femoral artery. At this site, a branch of the femoral vein crosses behind the proximal segment of the superficial femoral artery; thus, attempts at gaining arterial access might puncture both the artery and the vein creating a connection between the two vascular structures. An arteriovenous fistula manifests as a continuous bruit over the access site and is usually asymptomatic but may be associated with a hematoma. The diagnosis is confirmed by ultrasound. Iatrogenic arteriovenous fistulae lead to small and insignificant left-to-right shunts with no clinical consequence and a benign outcome. They close spontaneously in nearly 40% of cases; the remaining cases with persistence of the fistula usually remain asymptomatic and require no therapy (6). Rarely, the shunt may be large and create high-output failure or impair venous outflow and require surgical correction. An example of an arteriovenous fistula is shown in Video 3-5.

Rare vascular complications include arterial thrombosis, distal embolization, arterial dissection, and vessel perforation. These potentially serious complications occur more commonly in the presence of significant, underlying atherosclerotic peripheral vascular disease. The acute onset of pain, pallor, and pulselessness of an entire limb suggest thrombotic occlusion at the arterial access site; involvement of just the distal extremity is more consistent with distal embolization. Either complication may be caused by a thrombus introduced at the time of catheterization or during hemostasis, or from a clot developing at the puncture site (Video 3-6). In both situations, the manifestation of acute limb ischemia represents an emergency and requires immediate vascular surgery consultation. Arterial dissection is usually caused by careless technique when obtaining arterial access (Video 3-7). Typically, the operator notices sluggish or even nonpulsatile arterial blood return when the needle is passed into the artery. This indicates that the needle tip is partly subintimal. Guide-wire passage with the needle in this position dissects the artery. The complication is usually identified only when the operator notices resistance to wire passage or that the wire does not successfully achieve the central aorta. Fortunately, because the direction of the dissection is retrograde and against blood flow, most iatrogenic femoral artery or iliac dissections heal spontaneously and are of no clinical consequence. However, a large dissection flap may close the artery, causing acute limb ischemia. Vessel perforation is a highly unusual complication; it may occur from an excessively high puncture during attempts at gaining femoral access or when rigid catheters or sheaths are forcibly passed through tortuous, calcified, noncompliant iliac vessels.

Renal Failure. Renal failure is one of the more common complications of cardiac catheterization and is associated with increased morbidity and mortality (7). Using a definition of more than a 25% increase in baseline serum creatinine at 48 hours, the incidence of renal failure varies from less than 2% in the general population to as great as 30% for certain high-risk subgroups (8). These subgroups include patients with chronic renal insufficiency (estimated glomerular filtration rate <60 mL/min/1.7 m^2), diabetes, anemia, advanced (>75 years) age, heart failure, or shock at time of catheterization and hypovolemia. Volume of contrast is also an important risk factor. The low-osmolar contrast agents are associated with less nephropathy compared with high osmolality agents.

Although most cases of renal failure that occur after cardiac catheterization are due to contrast-induced nephropathy, it is important to consider other causes of renal failure. These include prerenal azotemia from a dehydrated state, cholesterol embolization syndrome, and nephrotoxicity caused by concomitant use of drugs such as angiotensin-converting enzyme inhibitors or nonsteroidal anti-inflammatory agents.

Careful patient selection and management before catheterization based on published guidelines help prevent contrast-induced nephropathy (7, 8). Patients at high risk for this complication should be adequately hydrated before the procedure with at least 1 L isotonic saline infused before and during the procedure with 100 to 150 mL/hr infused for at least 6 hours after the procedure. Some evidence supports the use of sodium bicarbonate infusion and N-acetylcysteine administration to prevent contrast-induced nephropathy. It is important to use only the minimum amount of contrast needed to perform the study. Contrast use can be minimized by avoiding left ventriculography if appropriate, performing staged procedures to accomplish coronary revascularization, and using biplane angiography suites.

Contrast Reactions. Two types of contrast reactions are described (9). *Immediate* reactions occur within an hour of contrast administration, typically manifesting in the cardiac catheterization laboratory or soon after the procedure. Immediate reactions are potentially serious and are often called *anaphylactoid* because of their similarity to anaphylaxis. They are termed *anaphylactoid* because these reactions are histamine mediated but are not IgE mediated like true anaphylaxis. A constellation of symptoms occur including nausea and vomiting, diffuse erythema, urticaria, angioedema, bronchospasm, laryngospasm, and hypotension; death from a contrast reaction is exceedingly rare (1 in 100,000). *Delayed* reactions occur 1 hour to 1 week after exposure. The mechanism of the delayed reactions is type IV hypersensitivity, and it manifests primarily as skin reactions (urticaria, maculopapular rash, erythema multiforme).

Patients with prior contrast reaction are at high risk for recurrence with subsequent exposure. Similarly, patients with a history of severe food or drug allergies and asthma are at increased risk. The relevance of seafood, shellfish, or iodine allergy in predicting contrast allergy is not clear and probably carries as much predictive value as a history of other food or drug allergy. Use of nonionic contrast is associated with lower incidence of contrast reactions in patients who previously experienced this complication with ionic contrast agents. Although most cardiac catheterization laboratories pretreat patients with a history of contrast allergy with systemic steroids (typical regimen: 40–60 mg prednisone 12 hours and 2 hours before contrast exposure), the value of pretreatment with steroids to prevent anaphylactoid reactions remains somewhat controversial. Notably, studies that show a lower incidence of contrast reactions administered steroids 12 hours and 2 hours before exposure; no effect was obtained from a single dose 2 hours before exposure. Furthermore, steroid pretreatment may reduce but does not eliminate the risk for a serious contrast reaction. Thus, the risks and benefits of contrast exposure in patients who have previously experienced a life-threatening reaction to contrast should be carefully considered. General principles and guidelines for treatment of immediate contrast reactions are outlined in Table 3-4 (9, 10).

Cholesterol Embolization. Cholesterol embolization is a rare but potentially lethal complication of catheterization. It is difficult to estimate its true incidence because subtle cases may not be diagnosed, and the manifestations may occur days to weeks after catheterization and not be attributed to the catheterization event. Some cases of renal failure after catheterization

Table 3-4.	Guidelines for Management of Contrast Reactions

Urticaria, Pruritus, and Erythema

Initial therapy
    Diphenhydramine 25–50 mg intravenously (IV)

If Severe and Not Responsive to Initial Therapy
    Epinephrine 0.1–0.3 mL of a 1:1,000 solution subcutaneously (SC) or intramuscularly
    (IM); repeat every 15 minutes up to 1 mL
    H2 blocker (cimetidine 300 mg or ranitidine 50 mg IV)

Bronchospasm

For mild reactions
    Oxygen by mask
    Inhaled bronchodilator if mild
    Diphenhydramine 50 mg IV
    H2 blocker (cimetidine 300 mg or ranitidine 50 mg IV)
    Hydrocortisone 200–400 mg IV

For more serious reactions
    All of above
    Epinephrine 0.1–0.3 mL of a 1:1,000 solution SC or IM; repeat every 15 minutes up
    to 1 mL

Facial Edema, Laryngospasm, or Laryngeal Edema

Oxygen by mask

Airway management (anesthesia)

Diphenhydramine 50 mg IV

H2 blocker (cimetidine 300 mg or ranitidine 50 mg IV)

Hydrocortisone 200–400 mg IV

Epinephrine 0.1–0.3 mL of a 1:1,000 solution SC or IM; repeat every 15 minutes up
to 1 mL

For more serious reactions, **epinephrine IV bolus 10 mg/min and infusion 1–4 mg/min**

Hypotension/Generalized Anaphylactoid Reaction

Intravenous fluids (normal saline)

Airway management/resuscitation team

Oxygen by mask

Diphenhydramine 50 mg IV

H2 blocker (cimetidine 300 mg or ranitidine 50 mg IV)

Hydrocortisone 200–400 mg IV

Epinephrine IV bolus 10 mg/min and infusion 1–4 mg/min

Dopamine (2–15 μg/Kg/min IV or phenylephrine to support blood pressure

---

may be from cholesterol embolization. The classic symptoms are livedo reticularis or "blue toe syndrome" (Fig. 3-3), renal failure, and eosinophilia. Systemic symptoms such as fever, myalgias, and a confusional state may develop together with ischemic bowel. The outcome of cholesterol embolization syndrome is often poor, and treatment is primarily supportive.

Miscellaneous and Unusual Complications from Cardiac Catheterization. A variety of unusual complications from catheterization procedures have been reported. These include local infection at the access site possibly leading to systemic sepsis, pyrogen reaction, catheter entrapment, air embolism, pulmonary artery rupture, cardiac perforation, pulmonary embolism or deep venous thrombosis, compartment syndrome, and nerve injury. Although these complications are unusual, all practicing invasive and interventional cardiologists should be aware of their existence. Cardiac perforation is a rare complication of catheterization; perforation of the left ventricle may arise from improper positioning of a catheter coupled with a power injector during performance of ventriculography (Video 3-8). Catheter entrapment may occur when a catheter is rotated in the presence of marked iliac tortuosity and a kink develops (Fig. 3-4). Sudden damping or loss of the catheter pressure should lead one to suspect kinking of the catheter. If this occurs, pulling back on the catheter may tighten the kink, creating a knot that prevents removal of the catheter. The sharp angle at the kink site may also injure the iliac artery. Furthermore, the kink leads to a weak spot in the catheter, and forceful tugging may avulse the catheter at the kink site. Successful removal involves careful rotation of the catheter in the direction opposite it was initially turned and careful passage of the guide wire.

Summary. Cardiac catheterization is associated with numerous potential complications. Although these cannot be entirely eliminated, the incidence of complications can be reduced by careful patient selection and preparation, and meticulous attention to detail. Furthermore, performance of these procedures by operators with clinical experience and great skill using proper technique also lead to improved patient outcomes.

References

1. Chandresakar B, Doucet S, Bilodeau L, et al: Complications of cardiac catheterization in the current era: A single-center experience. Catheter Cardiovasc Interv 2001;52:289–295.
2. Sankaranarayanan R, Msairi A, Davis G: Stroke following cardiac catheterization: A preventable and treatable complication. J Invasive Cardiol 2007;19:40–45.
3. Kent KC, Moscucci M, Mansour KA, et al: Retroperitoneal hematoma after cardiac catheterization: Prevalence, risk factors, and optimal management. J Vasc Surg 1994;20:905–913.
4. Sreeram S, Lumsden AB, Miller JS, et al: Retroperitoneal hematoma following femoral arterial catheterization: A serious and often fatal complication. Am Surg 1993;59:94–98.
5. Webber GW, Jang J, Gustavson S, Olin JW: Contemporary management of postcatheterization pseudoaneurysms. Circulation 2007;115:2666–2674.
6. Kelm M, Perings SM, Jax T, et al: Incidence and clinical outcome of iatrogenic femoral arteriovenous fistulas. Implications for risk stratification and treatment. J Am Coll Cardiol 2002;40:291–297.
7. Schweiger MJ, Chambers CE, Davidson CJ, et al: Prevention of contrast induced nephropathy: Recommendations for the high risk patient undergoing cardiovascular procedures. Catheter Cardiovasc Interv 2007;69:135–140.
8. Tepel M, Aspelin P, Lameire N: Contrast-induced nephropathy. A clinical and evidence-based approach. Circulation 2006;113:1799–1806.
9. Meth MJ, Maibach HI: Current understanding of contrast media reactions and implications for clinical management. Drug Safety 2006;29:133–141.
10. Goss JE, Chambers CE, Heupler FA: Systemic anaphylactoid reactions to iodinated contrast media during cardiac catheterization procedures: Guidelines for prevention, diagnosis and treatment. Cathet Cardiovasc Diagn 1995;34:99–104.

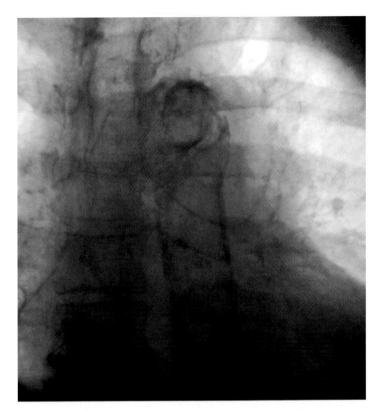

Figure 3-1. This fluoroscopic image was obtained in an 86-year-old woman undergoing coronary angiography and provides an example of dense calcification of the aorta associated with an increased risk for stroke during cardiac catheterization.

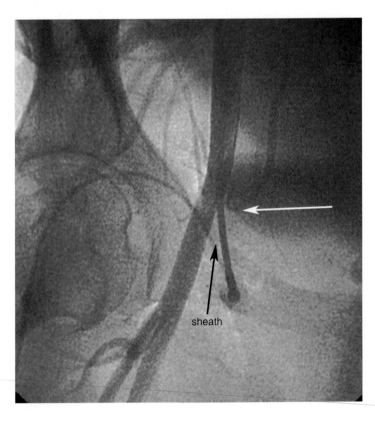

Figure 3-2. Femoral artery angiogram obtained in a patient undergoing cardiac catheterization. This is an example of a high stick with the sheath insertion site above the level of the inferior epigastric artery *(white arrow)*. This patient experienced development of a retroperitoneal hemorrhage after sheath removal that required 2 units of blood.

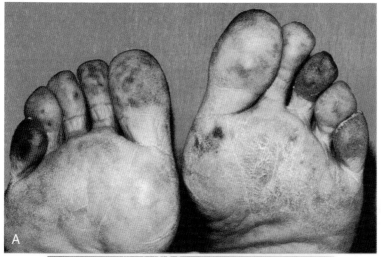

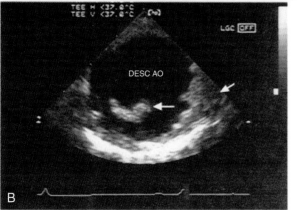

Figure 3-3. Example of "blue toes" caused by cholesterol embolization syndrome (A). Note the friable atheroma (arrows) in the descending aorta (DESC AO) as seen on transesophageal echo cardiography. (B). (From Pai RG, Heywood JT: Atheroembolism. Images in clinical medicine. N Engl J Med 1995;333:852, by permission.)

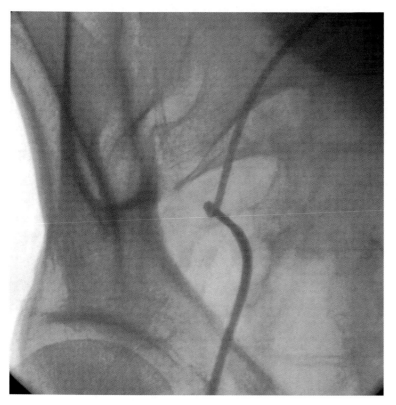

Figure 3-4. Presence of tortuous iliac arteries led to kinking of a right coronary catheter during attempts at selective coronary engagement. The kinked catheter can be difficult to disentangle, and the sharp ends of the kinked catheter may cause arterial injury.

RIGHT AND LEFT HEART CATHETERIZATION PART 1: PERFORMANCE OF RIGHT AND LEFT HEART CATHETERIZATION

Catheterization of the right and left side of the heart serve as the foundation of all catheter-based procedures including hemodynamic assessments, angiographic procedures, and cardiovascular interventions. Although the methods and equipment developed to perform these procedures have changed over the years, mastery of the durable principles underlying these techniques is essential for physicians regularly performing these procedures.

Commonly performed, nonselective angiographic procedures are left or right ventriculography, pulmonary angiography, and aortography (ascending, thoracic, or abdominal aorta). Selective angiographic procedures include native coronary, coronary bypass graft, and peripheral arterial angiography. These imaging procedures are routinely performed as part of the invasive evaluation for ischemic, myocardial, pericardial, valvular, peripheral vascular, and congenital heart disorders. Detailed descriptions and examples of these angiograms are provided in later sections.

Right and left heart catheterization are commonly performed to measure intracardiac pressures, cardiac outputs, and vascular resistances forming a discipline known as *hemodynamics*. A complete or partial hemodynamic assessment provides physiologic information that may be of great value in the diagnosis and management of patients with heart failure syndromes, pulmonary edema, shock, unexplained dyspnea, hypotension, respiratory failure, renal failure, peripheral edema, valvular heart disease, pericardial disease, hypertrophic cardiomyopathy, or congenital heart disease.

Cardiac catheterization is overall a safe procedure; the multiple, serious potential complications from right and left heart catheterization have been described. Inserting catheters into the left heart is frequently avoided in patients with known left ventricular thrombus or active aortic valve endocarditis to minimize the risk for embolization. Arrhythmias may arise from catheters placed in the right or left heart. Catheter placement in the right ventricular outflow tract can lead to right bundle branch block; left bundle branch block may arise when the aortic valve is crossed. Thus, patients with existing left bundle branch block may experience development of complete block when right heart catheterization is performed; similarly, patients with underlying right bundle branch block may experience development of complete heart block when the catheter crosses the aortic valve during a left heart catheterization. Normal conduction is generally restored with prompt removal of the offending catheter but may persist for some time and even require placement of a temporary pacemaker.

Equipment Choices. Angiography requires an appropriate catheter and a method to inject contrast. A pigtail catheter (end hole and numerous side holes) is commonly used in large, high-pressure structures such as the aorta or the left ventricle. Angiography of smaller, low-pressure structures, such as the pulmonary artery or the left ventricle, is often accomplished with a Berman catheter, a balloon flotation catheter similar to a Swann–Ganz catheter and constructed of multiple side holes near the tip but no end hole or thermistor. Selective angiography of vascular structures such as the coronary, cerebral, or visceral arteries requires specific catheters designed for those purposes. Contrast can be injected either by hand or by a power injector; hand injection is usually sufficient to image small vascular beds such as the coronary arteries. Power injectors are needed to adequately opacify large structures with high flow rates such as the aorta, pulmonary arteries, or ventricles.

Equipment needed for a hemodynamic evaluation includes a catheter, a transducer, fluid-filled tubing to connect the catheter to the transducer, and a physiologic recorder to display, analyze, print, and store the hemodynamic waveforms. End-hole catheters are used when sampling pressures within small chambers or when needed to identify pressure gradients over relatively small areas. The commonly used pig-tail catheter has an end hole and multiple side holes; this catheter is adequate if sampling pressure from a large, uniform chamber such as the aorta or left ventricle but will not have the required resolution to discern pressure gradients within the left ventricle. Catheters with an end hole and side holes at the tip prevent damping or artifactual waveforms because of positioning of the catheter tip against the chamber wall and are useful for collecting samples for oxygen saturation. The Swann–Ganz catheter is the most commonly used catheter for measuring right heart pressures. In addition to the balloon at the tip for flotation, it consists of an end hole (distal port), a side hole 30 cm from the catheter tip (proximal port), and a thermistor for measurement of thermodilution cardiac output. This catheter is used extensively in modern cardiac catheterization laboratories and at the bedside in intensive care units. Other catheters used for hemodynamic assessments include the balloon-wedge catheter (end hole but no thermistor), and the stiffer Layman and Cournand catheters (end hole), National Institutes of Health catheter (multiple side holes near the tip and no end hole), and the Goodale–Lubin catheter (end hole and two single side holes near the tip). Most catheterization laboratories use table-mounted, fluid-filled transducers. Under certain circumstances, pressure may be measured directly in the cardiac chamber or vessel by use of a tiny transducer (micromanometer) mounted at the tip of a catheter avoiding the limitations of a fluid-filled system. This is often the case when precise hemodynamic measurements are required as part of a research study; the most common clinical use is for measurement of intracoronary pressure and assessment of fractional flow reserve. A variety of proprietary computer systems are available for displaying, printing, analyzing, and storing hemodynamic waveforms.

Performance of Right Heart Catheterization. Performance of right heart catheterization is easily accomplished from the right internal jugular or subclavian veins using a balloon flotation catheter. Once access is obtained, a balloon flotation catheter is inserted to 20 cm and the balloon inflated. Attaching the catheter to a pressure transducer allows the operator to proceed using a pressure-guided technique that does not necessarily require fluoroscopy. Using this method, the operator advances the catheter with the balloon inflated and carefully watches the pressure waveforms change as the catheter tip enters each chamber. Pressure is recorded in the right atrium, right ventricle, and pulmonary artery. With the catheter positioned in the pulmonary artery, the operator measures thermodilution cardiac output and collects pulmonary artery blood for oximetric analysis to screen for a shunt and determine cardiac output by the Fick method. Finally, with the balloon inflated, the catheter is slowly advanced until a pulmonary capillary wedge pressure is obtained. Fluoroscopy is used when the pressure-guided technique does not allow successful catheter placement, a common occurrence when there is cardiac chamber enlargement.

Performing right heart catheterization from the femoral veins requires fluoroscopy. Because a substantial amount of catheter manipulation is often needed to pass the catheter into the pulmonary artery, the pressure transducer is not usually connected until the pulmonary artery is reached. The balloon is inflated just as the catheter exits the sheath. Under radiographic guidance, the catheter is advanced until it enters the right atrium (Fig. 4-1). From this location, a balloon flotation catheter readily crosses the tricuspid valve and enters the right ventricle. From here, however, advancing the catheter to the pulmonary artery may prove challenging. Beginning with the catheter tip approximately in the midportion of the right ventricle (Fig. 4-2), the operator aggressively rotates the catheter in a clockwise direction with the balloon inflated until the catheter tip points superiorly into the pulmonary artery outflow tract. Gently advancing the catheter from this position allows it to enter either the right or left pulmonary artery (Fig. 4-3). Some operators use a less elegant technique relying on a loop formed in the right atrium (Fig. 4-4). This positions the catheter so that simply advancing it with the balloon inflated allows the catheter to easily cross the tricuspid valve and enter the pulmonary outflow tract (Fig. 4-5). The relatively floppy Swan–Ganz catheter may be difficult to manipulate into the pulmonary artery or wedge position in the presence of pulmonary hypertension or severe tricuspid regurgitation. In such cases, catheter manipulation may be facilitated by stiffening the Swan–Ganz catheter with a 0.025-inch guide wire inserted into the distal lumen.

Performance of Left Heart Catheterization. Retrograde placement of a catheter from the aorta into the left ventricle is accomplished using a pigtail catheter prolapsed across the valve. This is performed by first advancing the pigtail catheter to the ascending aorta and positioning the catheter just above the aortic valve so that the loop of the pigtail appears like the number 6 (Fig. 4-6). The operator gently pushes the catheter onto the valve allowing the loop of the pigtail to slide up the aortic wall (Fig. 4-7). By gently pulling back on the catheter, the loop of the pigtail falls across the valve; at this point, the operator should gently slide the catheter forward to achieve its position in the left ventricle (Fig. 4-8). The catheter may need a gentle clockwise or counterclockwise turn to facilitate crossing the valve, or the catheter may need to be stiffened with a J-tipped guide wire, particularly if there is iliac or aortic tortuosity. The catheter position usually requires adjustment to avoid significant ectopy; the optimal position is in the midcavity of the ventricle in the left ventricular inflow tract just in front of the mitral valve.

Retrograde crossing of the aortic valve in a patient with aortic stenosis using the method of catheter prolapse rarely succeeds. One technique to cross a stenotic valve in a retrograde fashion utilizes a straight wire coupled with a catheter, systematically interrogating the valve to find the orifice. A 0.035-inch straight wire is loaded into a pigtail catheter and advanced until the tip exits the catheter and strikes the aortic valve annulus (Fig. 4-9). If this does not succeed in crossing the valve, then the tip of the straight wire is positioned at a location higher along the valve plane by advancing more of the pigtail catheter relative to the wire (Fig. 4-10). Again, the wire is systematically advanced from this location with several passes made. By making minor adjustments in the length of the pigtail catheter advanced relative to the tip of the straight wire, the wire tip can be systematically "walked" from back to front along a plane. If this does not successfully gain entry into the left ventricle, then the catheter is rotated clockwise or counterclockwise to change the orientation of the plane of the catheter, and again, the wire tip is "walked" from the back to the front of the annulus until the valve is crossed. The chances of crossing the valve are increased as the number of passes is increased. Sometimes, a pigtail catheter does not allow the wire to reach all areas of the valve plane. This is particularly true if the heart is horizontal because the valve plane will be oriented more vertically. When this occurs, other useful catheters include the Judkins right and the Judkins left (particularly the JL6 catheter), a multipurpose catheter, or a left Amplatz catheter.

Performance of Trans-septal Heart Catheterization. Entering the left ventricle via a retrograde approach is not always feasible, and some catheter-based procedures require access to the left atrium. Trans-septal catheterization is necessary in these situations. This procedure is often performed when it is necessary to measure left ventricular pressure or perform left ventriculography in the presence of a mechanical aortic valve or severe aortic stenosis. Another common indication includes the need to accurately measure left atrial pressure in a patient with mitral stenosis. Interventional procedures that require trans-septal puncture include mitral balloon valvuloplasty, percutaneous delivery of left atrial appendage exclusion devices, percutaneous mitral valve repairs, placement of a percutaneous left ventricular assist device, and some electrophysiologic procedures.

Performance of trans-septal puncture is technically demanding (1). The goal is to puncture the atrial septum at the fossa ovalis. It is important for the operator to understand the relevant anatomic relationships in both the anteroposterior and lateral radiographic projections to safely accomplish this. Biplane fluoroscopic imaging facilitates the procedure, allowing the operator to quickly check catheter position in both radiographic projections. Some operators routinely puncture the septum under guidance by intracardiac echocardiography, and some operators perform pulmonary angiography before the procedure relying on the levo phase to outline the location of the atrial septum. Relative contraindications to this procedure include the presence of coagulopathy, marked scoliosis, left atrial myxoma, left atrial thrombus, massive aortic dilatation, and thoracic deformity.

The puncture is accomplished with a Brockenbrough needle (Fig. 4-11) within a trans-septal sheath (usually about 60 cm long) and dilator. The procedure is performed from the right femoral vein; advancement and manipulation of the needle from the left femoral vein is not advised. Arterial access is obtained, and a pigtail catheter positioned on the aortic valve in the noncoronary cusp to allow identification of the aorta by fluoroscopy. Using an anteroposterior projection, the operator passes a 0.025-inch exchange length (cm) guide wire from the right femoral vein to the superior vena cava, and a 7 French trans-septal sheath and dilator positioned in the superior vena cave (Fig. 4-12). The wire is removed and the Brockenbrough needle inserted into the dilator taking care to keep the end of the needle well within the dilator (usually about 1 cm from the tip). The long metal needle has an obturator or stylet to prevent plugging or kinking; this should remain in place as the needle is advanced and then removed when the end of the needle approaches the tip of the dilator. As the needle is advanced from the femoral vein to the superior vena cava, it should be allowed to freely rotate within the dilator and never be forcibly advanced. The proximal end of the needle is attached to a three-way stopcock allowing the ability to monitor pressure and inject contrast or saline. At this point, biplane fluoroscopy using the anteroposterior and straight lateral projections helps position the needle for the septal puncture.

Positioning the needle properly is critical to success. The hub end of the Brockenbrough needle has an arrow that points in the same direction as the curve of the needle tip. This relation is important. The entire unit consisting of the sheath, dilator, and needle is rotated clockwise using the anteroposterior fluoroscopic projection so that the tip points toward the patient's left. The entire apparatus is slowly withdrawn from the superior vena cava and the operator senses a series of "bumps" associated with leftward movement of the dilator tip. The first occurs when the catheter enters the right atrium at the crista terminalis, a second one occurs as the catheter tip passes over the ascending aorta, and the third when it enters the fossa ovalis. The arrow at the needle hub should be pointed slightly posterior and to the left, identified as the 4-o'clock position by the arrow (the ceiling represents 12 o'clock and the floor 6 o'clock). The tip of the catheter should be clearly below the aortic annulus. If the correct position is confirmed, the needle can be advanced out the tip of the dilator and a small amount of contrast injected to stain the septum (Fig. 4-13). The puncture can be made at this location by advancing only the needle while the proximal end of the needle is attached to a pressure transducer. Confirmation that the needle tip is within the left atrium relies on the demonstration of a left atrial pressure waveform and oxygen saturation greater than 90%. Once the operator has successfully entered the left atrium with the needle tip, the needle is fixed in that position and the dilator advanced so that the tip of the dilator is within the left atrium. The needle is gently removed and replaced with a 0.025-inch J-tipped guide wire. The guide wire is advanced until it is secure within the left atrium or passes into a pulmonary vein, and the dilator and sheath advanced over the wire until the tip of the sheath is within the left atrium (Fig. 4-14). The wire and dilator are removed leaving the sheath within the left atrium (Fig. 4-15). The sheath is carefully aspirated and flushed with heparinized saline. At this point, many operators administer systemic heparin. Left atrial pressure is recorded. A balloon flotation catheter (Berman) can be advanced through the trans-septal sheath across the mitral valve to measure left ventricular pressure or perform left ventriculography; simultaneous left ventricular and left atrial pressure can be measured by recording pressure from the side arm of the trans-septal sheath (left atrial pressure) and the end of the Berman catheter (left ventricle) allowing assessment of the mitral valve gradient. The aortic valve gradient can be determined by simultaneously recording pressure from the Berman catheter within the left ventricle and from a pigtail catheter in the aorta placed just above the valve.

References

1. Roelke M, Smith C, Palacios IF: The technique and safety of transseptal left heart catheterization: The Massachusetts General Hospital experience with 1279 procedures. Catheter Cardiovasc Diagn 1994;32:332–339.
2. Brockenbrough EC, Braunwald E, Ross J: Transseptal left heart catheterization: A review of 450 studies and description of improved technic. Circulation 1962;25:15–21.

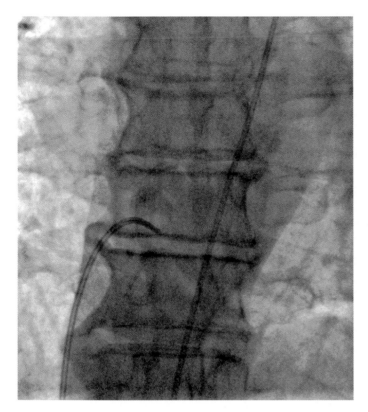

FIGURE 4-1. Anteroposterior projection demonstrating the technique for positioning the Swann–Ganz catheter into the right heart from the femoral vein. The catheter tip is within the right atrium.

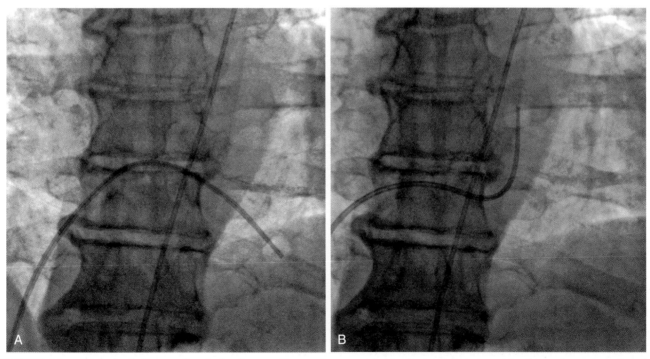

FIGURE 4-2. With the balloon inflated, the Swann–Ganz catheter is advanced across the tricuspid valve and positioned to the left of the spine in the outflow tract (*A*). The catheter should not be advanced to the apex of the right ventricle because this will make it more difficult to turn into the outflow tract. From this position, the catheter is aggressively turned in a clockwise manner with the balloon inflated until the tip points up and into the pulmonary outflow tract (*B*).

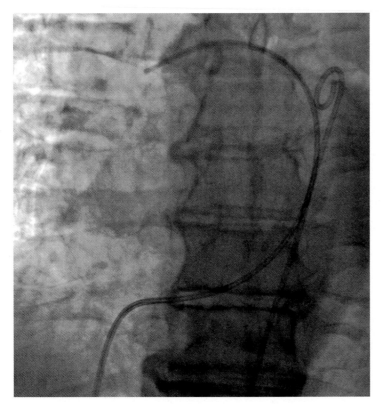

FIGURE 4-3. Final position of the Swan–Ganz catheter in the pulmonary artery from the femoral vein.

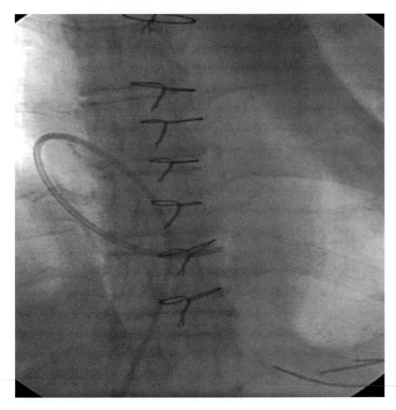

FIGURE 4-4. Another technique used to pass the Swann–Ganz catheter from the femoral vein uses a backward loop created in the right atrium. From this position, the catheter can be easily advanced with the balloon inflated and often points directly to the outflow tract after passing the tricuspid valve.

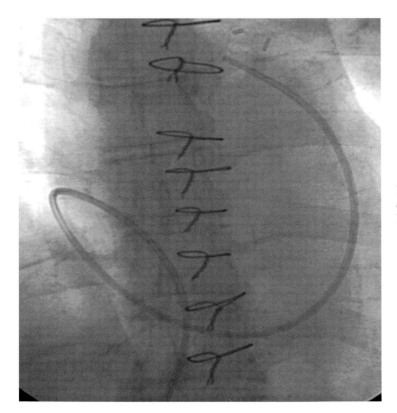

FIGURE 4-5. Final position of the Swann–Ganz catheter in the pulmonary artery using the backward loop technique.

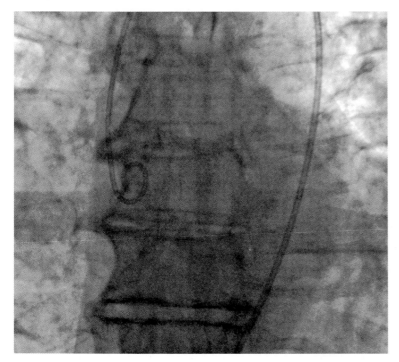

FIGURE 4-6. Technique for prolapsing a pigtail catheter across the aortic valve. The catheter is first advanced above the aortic valve and positioned to look like the number 6 as shown here.

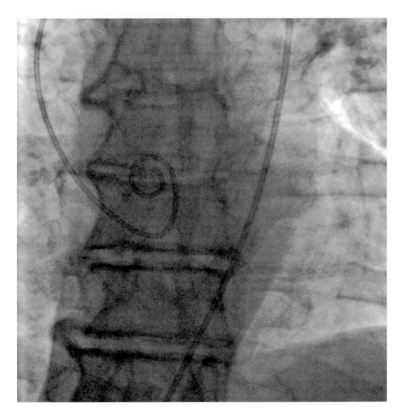

FIGURE 4-7. Technique for prolapsing a pigtail catheter across the aortic valve. Once the catheter is positioned as shown in Figure 4-6, the catheter is pushed forward, allowing it to ride up the aorta as shown here. This may result in prolapse across the valve; however, usually, the catheter must next be gently drawn back, thereby allowing the catheter to advance across the valve. Once it advances across the valve, it often needs additional advancement to achieve the proper position within the left ventricle.

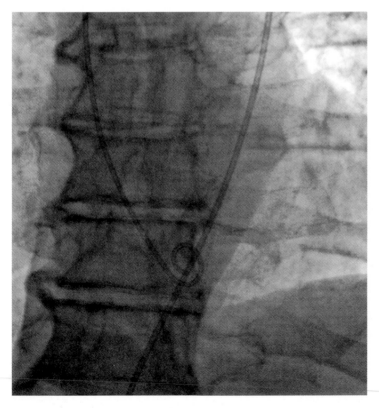

FIGURE 4-8. Technique for prolapsing a pigtail catheter across the aortic valve. The catheter has advanced across the aortic valve and is positioned in a stable location within the left ventricle.

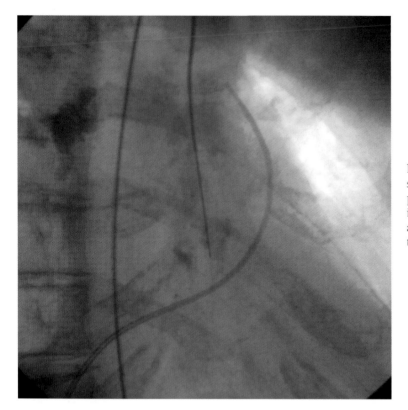

FIGURE 4-9. Straight-wire technique for crossing a stenotic aortic valve. The 0.035-inch guide wire is positioned within a pigtail catheter. The wire is pointing at the starting position, and is withdrawn and advanced within the catheter several times in an effort to cross the valve.

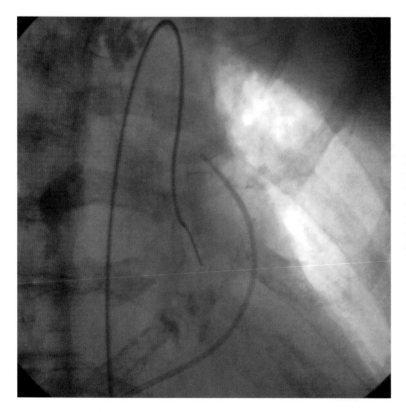

FIGURE 4-10. Straight-wire technique for crossing a stenotic aortic valve. If the initial position is unsuccessful, the pigtail catheter is advanced, providing access to a higher position on the valve. Varying the length of the pigtail catheter relative to the wire allows the operator to "walk" up and down the valve until successful.

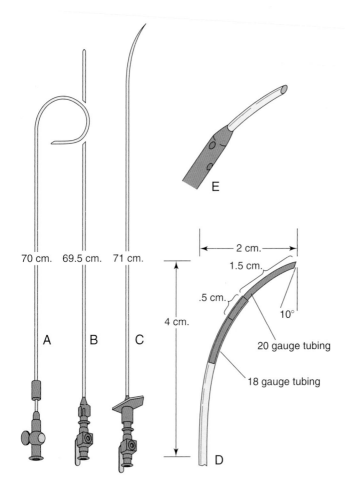
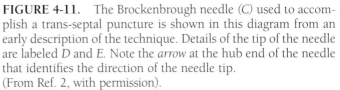

70 cm.   69.5 cm.   71 cm.

A   B   C

2 cm.

1.5 cm.

.5 cm.

4 cm.

10°

20 gauge tubing

18 gauge tubing

D

E

FIGURE 4-11. The Brockenbrough needle (*C*) used to accomplish a trans-septal puncture is shown in this diagram from an early description of the technique. Details of the tip of the needle are labeled *D* and *E*. Note the *arrow* at the hub end of the needle that identifies the direction of the needle tip.
(From Ref. 2, with permission).

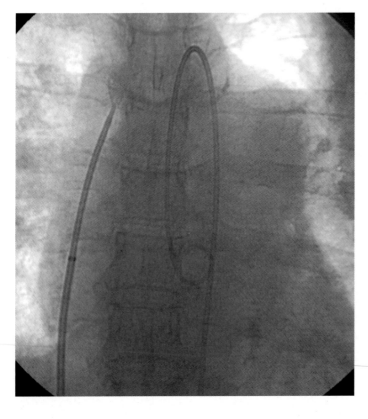

FIGURE 4-12. The sheath and dilator are first positioned in the superior vena cava as shown here to perform trans-septal puncture.

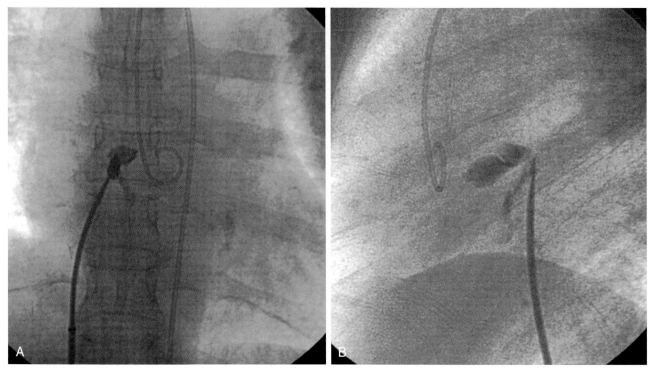

FIGURE 4-13. When the sheath, dilator, and needle assembly have reached the fossa ovalis, the needle may be gently advanced and the septum stained with contrast as shown here. *A,* Anteroposterior view. *B,* Lateral projection. Note location and orientation of the needle tip relative to the pigtail catheter placed on top of the aortic valve. The needle tip is facing posterior and below the aortic annulus.

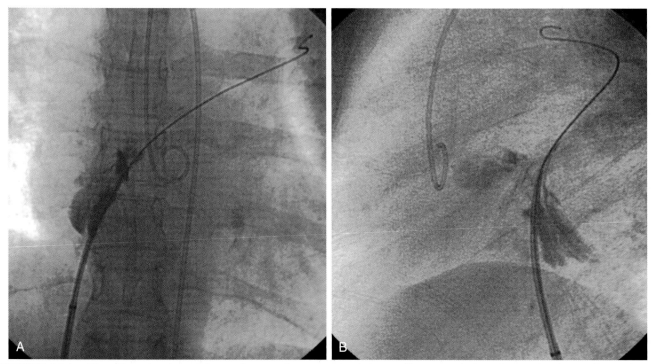

FIGURE 4-14. The dilator has been advanced across the septum and the needle removed. A guide wire has been advanced into a pulmonary vein to facilitate passage of the sheath and dilator. *A,* Anteroposterior view. *B,* Lateral projection.

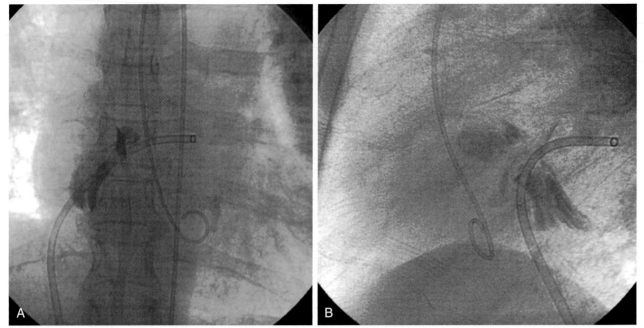

FIGURE 4-15.   Final position of the trans-septal sheath within the left atrium. *A*, Anteroposterior view. *B*, Lateral projection.

CHAPTER 5

RIGHT AND LEFT HEART CATHETERIZATION PART 2: COLLECTING AND ANALYZING HEMODYNAMIC DATA

Hemodynamic evaluation is an important and often overlooked component of cardiac catheterization. Obtaining sloppy, poor-quality information or misinterpreting waveforms can lead to major errors in diagnosis and management. Adopting a systematic approach to the collection, analysis, and interpretation of hemodynamic data improves procedural quality and reduces the potential for error.

Collection of Hemodynamic Waveforms. Nearly all clinical cardiac catheterization laboratories use disposable, fluid-filled transducers to measure pressure. These table-mounted transducers are calibrated in the factory but require balancing or "zeroing" before any measurements can be made. Balancing a transducer establishes a reference point for all subsequent pressure measurements. The "zero" position (also called the *phlebostatic axis*) indicates the level of the right atrium and is located at the patient's midchest in the anteroposterior dimension at the level of the sternal angle of Louis (4th intercostals space). A table-mounted transducer is placed at this level, opened to air, and set to zero. Inaccuracies in transducer position may lead to errors. For example, a transducer placed *above* the correct zero position furnishes a measured pressure *lower* than the actual pressure, whereas a transducer placed *below* the correct zero position results in a *higher* than actual pressure. During the case, the operator should be aware of the potential for transducer "drift" indicating either the loss of calibration or the loss of balance after initially setting the zero level.

Protocol for Collecting Hemodynamic Waveforms. Once the transducer is zeroed, data collection may begin. Following a routine protocol during a right and left heart catheterization prevents errors of omission (Table 5-1). After obtaining access, the physician positions the right heart catheter in the pulmonary artery and a pigtail catheter in the aorta. Cardiac output is measured using the thermodilution method. Blood is collected from the aorta and pulmonary artery for determination of oxygen saturation both to calculate cardiac output by the Fick method and to screen for the presence of a left-to-right intracardiac shunt. Aortic and pulmonary artery pressures are measured and the pigtail catheter advanced in a retrograde fashion across the aortic valve and into the left ventricle. The right heart catheter is advanced to the pulmonary capillary wedge position, and simultaneous left ventricular and pulmonary capillary wedge pressure (PCWP) are measured to screen for the presence of mitral stenosis. Pressure waveforms are recorded from each chamber as the right-sided catheter is withdrawn with careful attention paid as the catheter crosses the pulmonic and tricuspid

Table 5-1. **Components of a Routine Complete Right and Left Heart Catheterization**

a. Position pulmonary artery (PA) catheter

b. Position aortic (AO) catheter

c. Measure PA and AO pressure

d. Measure thermodilution cardiac output

e. Measure oxygen saturation in PA and AO blood samples to determine Fick output and screen for shunt

f. Enter the left ventricle (LV) by retrograde crossing of the AO valve

g. Advance PA catheter to pulmonary capillary wedge position (PCWP)

h. Measure simultaneous LV-PCWP to screen for mitral stenosis

i. Pullback from PCWP to PA

j. Pullback from PA to right ventricle (RV) to screen for pulmonic stenosis and record RV

k. Record simultaneous LV-RV to determine constrictive physiology

l. Pullback from RV to right atrium (RA) to screen for tricuspid stenosis and record RA

m. LV-AO pullback to screen for aortic stenosis

valves to screen for stenosis across these valves. Simultaneous right ventricular and left ventricular pressure recordings are obtained to screen for restrictive/constrictive physiology. The final maneuver consists of withdrawal of the pigtail catheter from the left ventricle into the aorta to screen for aortic valve stenosis.

Analysis and Interpretation of Hemodynamic Waveforms. Proper interpretation of pressure waveforms requires a consistent and systematic approach. The operator should first confirm the zero level, the scale of the recording, and the recording sweep speed. Data collection should follow a standard protocol as described earlier. Analysis of the data begins by critically assessing the waveforms and looking for high-fidelity tracings without overdamping or underdamping. Proper interpretation also requires a high-quality electrocardiographic tracing, and each pressure event should be timed with events on the ECG. Respiratory variation commonly affects right heart pressures. The operator should report pressures at end expiration. Finally, the operator should review the tracings for common artifacts that might lead to misinterpretation.

Normal Right Atrial Waveform. The normal right atrial pressure is 2 to 6 mm Hg with "a" and "v" waves and "x" and "y" descents (Fig. 5-1). The "a" wave represents the pressure increase within the right atrium caused by atrial contraction and follows the P wave on the electrocardiogram by about 80 milliseconds. The "x" descent represents the pressure decay after the "a" wave and reflects both atrial relaxation and the sudden downward motion of the atrioventricular junction occurring because of ventricular systole. A "c" wave is sometimes observed after the "a" wave from motion of the tricuspid annulus toward the right atrium at the onset of ventricular systole. The "c" wave follows the "a" wave by the same time as the PR interval on the electrocardiogram; first-degree atrioventricular block results in a more obvious "c" wave. When a "c" wave is present, the pressure decay after it is called an "x^1" descent. The "v" wave is due to passive venous filling of the atrium representing atrial diastole. Increased filling of the right atrium results in a prominent "v" wave. The peak of the right atrial "v" wave occurs at the end of ventricular systole when the atria are maximally filled and corresponds with the end of the T wave on the surface electrocardiogram. The pressure decay occurring after the "v" wave is the "y" descent and is due to rapid emptying of the right atrium when the tricuspid valve opens.

Normal Right Ventricular Waveform. Normal right ventricular systolic pressure is 20 to 30 mm Hg, and normal right ventricular end-diastolic pressure is 0 to 8 mm Hg. A normal right ventricular waveform is shown in Figure 5-2 and exhibits a rapid pressure increase and decline with ventricular contraction and relaxation. Early diastolic pressure is low and increases gradually to an end-diastolic pressure. With atrial contraction, an "a" wave may appear on the ventricular waveform at end diastole indicating reduced compliance of the right ventricle.

Normal Pulmonary Artery Waveform. Pulmonary artery systolic pressure is normally the same as right ventricular systolic pressure (20–30 mm Hg) with a diastolic pressure of 4 to 12 mm Hg (Fig. 5-3). The pulmonary artery pressure waveform increases rapidly toward a systolic peak. During the pressure decay there is a well-defined dicrotic notch from pulmonic valve closure and a diastolic trough. Peak systolic pressure occurs within the T wave on the surface electrocardiogram.

Normal Pulmonary Capillary Wedge Pressure Waveform. The pressure waveforms obtained from an end-hole catheter obstructing anterograde flow in the pulmonary artery reflect left atrial pressure. This is known as the *pulmonary capillary wedge pressure* (PCWP), and is usually obtained by inflating the balloon on a Swan–Ganz catheter in the pulmonary artery obstructing flow and "wedging" the catheter, creating a continuous column of fluid from the left atrium, to the pulmonary veins, pulmonary capillary bed, and pulmonary artery. A normal PCWP consists of "a" and "v" waves and "x" and "y" descents; the normal mean pressure is 2 to 14 mm Hg (Fig. 5-4). The PCWP tracing exhibits several important differences from a directly measured atrial pressure waveform. The "c" wave sometimes identified in an atrial waveform is absent because of the damped nature of the pressure wave. Because the pressure wave is transmitted through the pulmonary capillary bed, a significant time delay occurs between an electrocardiographic event and the onset of the corresponding pressure wave. Typically, the peak of the "a" wave follows the P wave on the electrocardiogram by about 240 milliseconds rather than 80 milliseconds as seen in the right atrial tracing. Similarly, the peak of the "v" wave occurs after the T wave has already been inscribed on the electrocardiogram.

Obtaining an accurate and high-quality PCWP tracing is not always easy or possible, particularly if pulmonary hypertension exists. Characteristics confirming a true PCWP include the presence of well-defined "a" and "v" waves and obtaining an oxygen saturation greater than 90% from the catheter tip when in the PCWP position.

Normal Left Ventricular Waveform. Normal left ventricular systolic pressure is 90 to 140 mm Hg, and normal end-diastolic pressure is 10 to 16 mm Hg. The left ventricular waveform is characterized by a rapid upstroke during ventricular contraction followed by rapid pressure decay during relaxation (Fig. 5-5). Pressure in early diastole is low and slowly increases until end diastole. Similar to the right ventricular waveform, an "a" wave may be seen in the left ventricular tracing at end diastole; however, this is usually abnormal and implies a noncompliant left ventricle. Left ventricular end-diastolic pressure is defined as the pressure just after the "a" wave and before the abrupt increase in systolic pressure coinciding with ventricular ejection.

Normal Central Aortic Pressure Waveform. Normal aortic systolic pressure is 90 to 140 mm Hg, and normal diastolic pressure is 60 to 90 mm Hg. Central aortic waveforms have a rapid upstroke, a systolic peak, and a clearly defined dicrotic notch because of closure of the aortic valve during pressure decay (Fig. 5-6). The peak systolic pressure equals the peak left ventricular systolic pressure unless there is obstruction within the left ventricle, at the aortic valve, or within the proximal aorta. The central aortic pressure waveform is composed of two components: the pressure wave generated from forward flow from left ventricular ejection plus the summation of pressure waves generated from "reflected" waves. The impact of reflected waves is more apparent the farther pressure is sampled from the aortic valve but is usually negligible. Under some circumstances, reflected waves may be significant. Reflected waves are increased in patients with aortic regurgitation, systemic hypertension, increased aortic stiffness, or peripheral vascular disease. The effect of reflected waves is particularly notable in peripheral arterial waveforms (brachial, femoral, and radial) and results in the phenomenon of "peripheral amplification" in which the peak systolic pressure exceeds central aortic pressure by 10 to 20 mm Hg (Fig. 5-7).

Simultaneous Measurement of Left and Right Ventricular Pressures. Simultaneous measurement of left and right ventricular pressures is performed to screen for the presence of restrictive or constrictive physiology and should be a part of all complete, hemodynamic evaluations. Fairly complex interactions occur between the cardiac chambers, the pericardium, and the intrathoracic cavity during the respiratory cycle. In general, in patients without constrictive physiology, the net effect of these interactions causes left and right ventricular diastolic pressures to differ by at least 5 mm Hg with variation during the respiratory cycle (Fig. 5-8A). Peak systolic pressure changes during inspiration and expiration in the right and left ventricle normally parallel each other (see Fig. 5-8B). One of the classic hemodynamic hallmarks of constrictive pericarditis can be demonstrated in simultaneously obtained right and left ventricular pressures where the finding of ventricular interdependence can be seen. This is manifest by the occurrence of the nadir of right ventricular systolic pressure at the peak left ventricular systolic pressure (1).

The impact of conduction abnormalities on hemodynamics is reflected in simultaneous right and left ventricular pressure tracings. Normally, the right ventricular waveform sits within the confines of the left ventricular wave (Fig. 5-9A). A right bundle branch block delays right ventricular contraction relative to left ventricular contraction, resulting in a delay in the right ventricular pressure wave and a shift to the right (see Fig. 5-9B). The opposite occurs with a left bundle branch block (see Fig. 5-9C).

Simultaneous Measurement of Pulmonary Capillary Wedge (or Left Atrial) and Left Ventricular Pressures. Simultaneous measurement of pulmonary capillary wedge (or left atrial) and left ventricular pressures specifically screens for mitral valve stenosis and is necessary to collect the data required for calculation of mitral valve orifice area in patients with known mitral stenosis. Normally, there should be no gradient between PCWP and left ventricular end-diastolic pressure (Fig. 5-10). A small gradient may be discernable only early in diastole. The time delay associated with the PCWP tracing causes the "a" and "v" waves to appear later in the left ventricular waveform and may be confused with a diastolic gradient in the presence of a large "v" wave. During simultaneous measurement of left atrial and left ventricular waveforms, the true position of the "v" wave can be appreciated; the "y" descent correlates with the decay in left ventricular pressure (Fig. 5-11). Thus, in the presence of a large "v" wave on the PCWP, the time delay can be corrected by shifting the PCWP to the left.

Simultaneous Measurement of Central Aorta and Left Ventricular Pressures. Simultaneous left ventricular and central aortic pressures are recorded in cases of known or suspected aortic stenosis to measure the transvalvular gradient and calculate aortic valve area. There are several ways to measure the gradient (2). The most accurate, but least practical, is to place one catheter above the aortic valve and another below the aortic valve via a transseptal approach. The easiest, most clinically practical, and most accurate method uses a dual-lumen catheter placed across the valve to measure simultaneous left ventricular and aortic pressures (Fig. 5-12). Simultaneous left ventricular and femoral arterial sheath pressures introduce substantial error into this measurement and should not be used for this purpose.

Hemodynamic Calculations. Several calculations are routinely made in conjunction with hemodynamic measurements obtained in the cardiac catheterization laboratory. These include the Fick method for determining cardiac output, calculation of resistances, and the calculation of orifice areas. Most of the commercially available, computerized hemodynamic data collection systems currently in use automatically calculate these values. The formulae for these calculations are provided in Table 5-2.

Potential Errors and Artifacts in Hemodynamic Determinations. Common errors in the collection and interpretation of hemodynamic data are listed in Table 5-3. These may lead to misdiagnosis or patient mismanagement. Some of the most commonly observed artifacts relate to an improper degree of damping. The *overdamped* tracing (Fig. 5-13) indicates the

Table 5-2.	Frequently Used Hemodynamic Formulae

I. Calculation of Cardiac Output by the Fick Method

$$\text{Cardiac output} = \frac{\text{oxygen consumption}}{(\text{arteriovenous oxygen difference}) \times (\text{hemoglobin}) \times 13.6}$$

where *oxygen consumption* = measured or assumed as 125 mL/min/m^2 for average individuals and 110 mL/min/m^2 for elderly patients; *arteriovenous oxygen difference* = arterial oxygen saturation − mixed venous oxygen saturation; *Hemoglobin* = hemoglobin concentration in g/dL; and *13.6* = a constant derived from the amount of oxygen carried per gram of hemoglobin (1.36 mL oxygen per gram of hemoglobin) times 10 to correct the units.

II. Calculation of Pulmonary Vascular Resistance (PVR)

$$\text{PVR} = \frac{(\text{mean pulmonary artery pressure}) - (\text{mean wedge pressure})}{\text{cardiac output}}$$

where *mean pulmonary artery pressure* and *mean wedge pressure* are in millimeters of mercury (mm Hg), and *cardiac output* is measured in liters per minute. This calculation will provide resistance in Woods units; multiplying this value by 80 converts Woods units to dynes/sec/cm^5; a normal pulmonary vascular resistance is roughly 70 dynes/sec/cm^5.

III. Calculation of Systemic Vascular Resistance (SVR)

$$\text{SVR} = \frac{(\text{mean aortic pressure}) - (\text{mean right atrial pressure})}{\text{cardiac output}}$$

where *mean aortic pressure* and *mean right atrial pressure* are measured in millimeters of mercury (mm Hg), and *cardiac output* is measured in liters per minute. This calculation will provide resistance in Woods units; multiplying this value by 80 converts Woods units to dynes/sec/cm^5. To calculate the systemic vascular resistance index, substitute the cardiac index for cardiac output in the formula; therefore, the systemic vascular resistance index (SVRI) formula is:

$$\text{SVRI} = (\text{SVR}) \times (\text{body surface area})$$

The normal SVR = 1170 ± 270 dynes/sec/cm^{-5}, and the normal SVRI = 2130 ± 450 dynes/sec/cm$^{-5} \times$ M^2

IV. Calculation of Mitral Valve Area (Based on Gorlin's Formula)

$$\text{Mitral valve area} = \frac{\text{cardiac output}}{(\text{diastolic filling period})(\text{heart rate})(37.9)(\sqrt{\text{pressure gradient}})}$$

where *cardiac output* is measured in milliliters per minute (mL/min); *diastolic filling period* is measured in seconds; *heart rate* is measured in beats per minute; *37.9* = the Gorlin's constant for the mitral valve; and $\sqrt{\text{pressure gradient}}$ = square root of the mean left ventricular-left atrial diastolic pressure gradient in millimeters of mercury (mm Hg).

V. Calculation of Aortic Valve Area (Based on Gorlin's Formula)

$$\text{Aortic valve area} = \frac{\text{cardiac output}}{\text{heart rate}(\text{SEP})(44.5)(\sqrt{\text{pressure gradient}})}$$

where *cardiac output* is measured in milliliters per minute (mL/min); *SEP* is the systolic ejection period in seconds; *heart rate* is measured in beats per minute; *44.5* = the Gorlin's constant for the aortic valve; and $\sqrt{\text{pressure gradient}}$ = square root of the mean left ventricular-aortic systolic pressure gradient in millimeters of mercury (mm Hg).

presence of excessive friction absorbing the force of the pressure wave somewhere in the line from the catheter tip to the transducer. The tracing lacks proper fidelity, and appears smooth and rounded. This artifact is usually caused by air bubbles in the tubing, catheter, or transducer, or a loose connection anywhere in the system. A thrombus or kink in the catheter may also cause this artifact. Underdamping causes "overshoot" or "ring" artifact (Fig. 5-14). This artifact manifests as one or more narrow "spikes" overshooting the true pressure during the systolic pressure increase with similar, negatively directed waves overshooting the true pressure contour during the downstroke. Tiny air bubbles oscillating rapidly back and forth cause this artifact and can be easily corrected by flushing the catheter or transducer. An appearance similar to overshoot or ring artifact is "catheter whip" or "fling" artifact. This artifact is created by acceleration of the fluid within the catheter from rapid catheter motion and is commonly

Table 5-3.	Common Sources of Error or Inaccuracy in Hemodynamic Assessment

1. Improper zero level or transducer balancing

2. Air bubbles, clot, or kinks in the system

3. Loose connections

4. Defective transducers

5. Tachycardia and loss of frequency response

6. Mechanical ventilators and excessive intrathoracic pressure changes

7. Artifacts:
   a. Overdamping
   b. Overshoot or "ring" artifact
   c. Catheter whip or "fling"
   d. Catheter entrapment
   e. Hybrid waveforms

seen with balloon-tipped catheters in hyperdynamic hearts or balloon-tipped catheters placed in the pulmonary artery with extraneous loops. Similar to ring artifact, catheter whip causes overestimation of the systolic pressure and underestimation of the diastolic pressure. This artifact is difficult to remedy; eliminating extra loops or deflation of the balloon can improve the appearance and limit this artifact.

Catheter malposition creates additional artifacts. *Catheter entrapment artifact* may be observed when measuring left ventricular pressure with an end-hole catheter, particularly in patients with severe left ventricular hypertrophy. If the tip of the catheter becomes buried or "entrapped" within the myocardium, it will reflect intramural rather than intracavitary pressure, resulting in a bizarre, spiked appearance to the left ventricular waveform (Fig. 5-15). A *hybrid tracing* results when the sampled pressure represents a mixture of the waveforms from more than one cardiac chamber. Hybrid tracings are commonly observed when a pigtail catheter with its multiple side holes straddles two cardiac chambers. The pressure waveform conveyed to the transducer contains pressure elements from each chamber. For example, a pigtail may be improperly positioned within the left ventricle with side holes lying above and below the aortic valve. The pressure waveform contains both aortic and left ventricular pressure waveform elements creating a "hybrid" of both chambers (Fig. 5-16). Hybrid tracings may also be observed during attempts at obtaining a PCWP particularly if pulmonary hypertension exists. In this case, the catheter may not completely occlude the pulmonary artery; the resulting waveform represents a mixture of a pulmonary artery and pulmonary capillary waveforms giving a falsely high value to the wedge pressure.

References

1. Hurrell DG, Nishimura RA, Higano ST, et al: Value of dynamic respiratory changes in left and right ventricular pressures for the diagnosis of constrictive pericarditis. Circulation 1996;93:2007–2013.
2. Fusman B, Faxon D, Feldman T: Hemodynamic rounds: Transvalvular pressure gradient measurement. Catheter Cardiovasc Interv 2001;53:553–561.

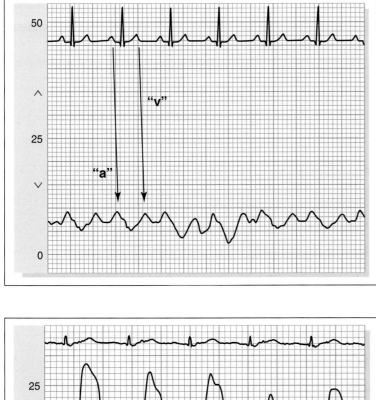

FIGURE 5-1. Normal right atrial waveform showing the timing of the "a" and "v" waves relative to the electrocardiogram.

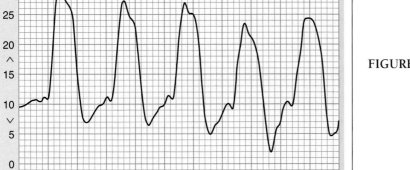

FIGURE 5-2. Normal right ventricular waveform.

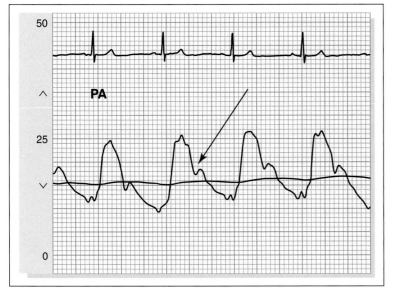

FIGURE 5-3. Normal pulmonary artery (PA) waveform with the *arrow* depicting the dicrotic notch.

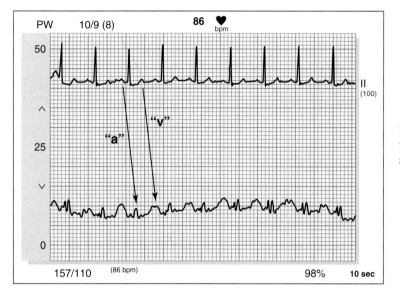
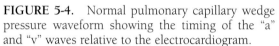

FIGURE 5-4.   Normal pulmonary capillary wedge pressure waveform showing the timing of the "a" and "v" waves relative to the electrocardiogram.

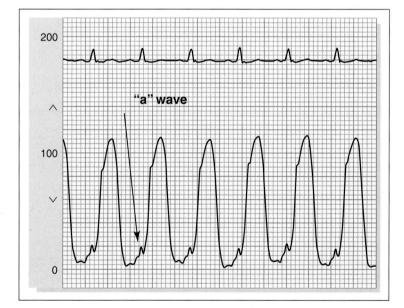

FIGURE 5-5.   Left ventricular waveform with a prominent "a" wave.

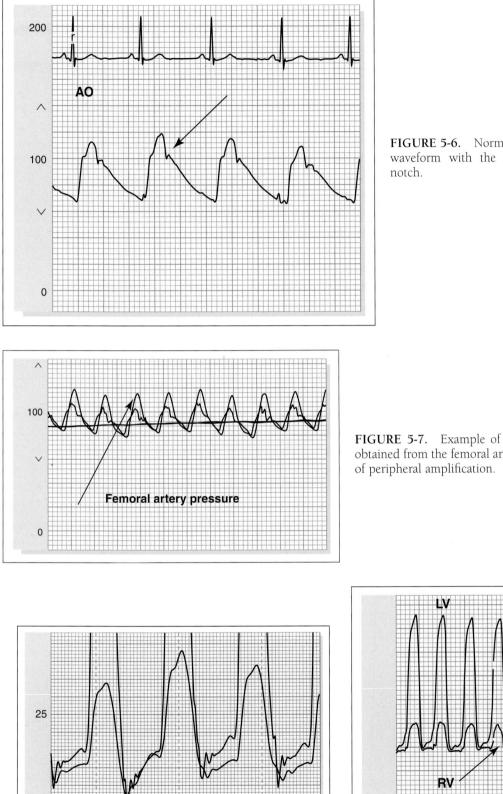

FIGURE 5-6. Normal central aortic (AO) pressure waveform with the *arrow* depicting the dicrotic notch.

FIGURE 5-7. Example of a peripheral artery waveform obtained from the femoral artery showing the phenomenon of peripheral amplification.

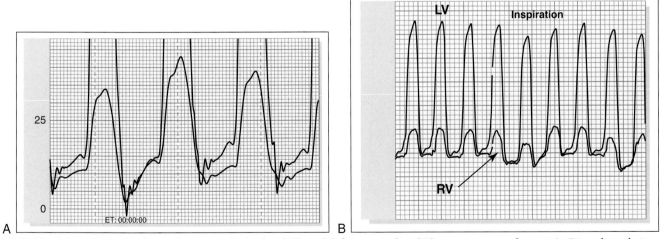

FIGURE 5-8. Normal relation between the right (RV) and left ventricular (LV) pressure waveforms. A, Diastolic relation. B, Systolic relation.

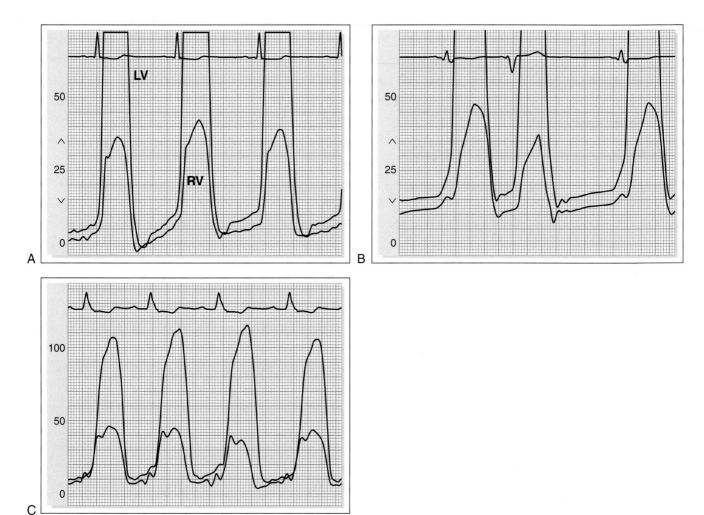

FIGURE 5-9. Effect of conduction abnormalities on simultaneous right (RV) and left ventricular (LV) pressure waveforms. Normally, the right ventricular pressure wave sits within the left ventricular pressure contour (A). In the presence of a right bundle branch block, the right ventricular wave is shifted to the right (B). Note how a premature ventricular contraction returns the right ventricular tracing to a more normal appearance. A left bundle branch block or intraventricular conduction delay interrupts left ventricular contraction relative to the right ventricle causing the right ventricular waveform to shift to the left (C).

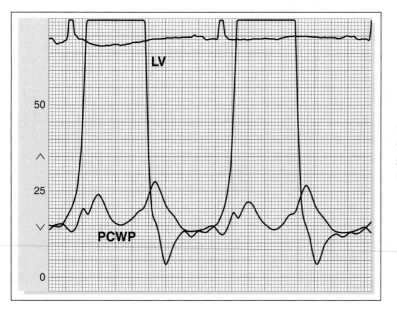

FIGURE 5-10. Normal simultaneous left ventricular (LV) and pulmonary capillary wedge pressure (PCWP) waveforms; this maneuver is performed to screen for mitral stenosis.

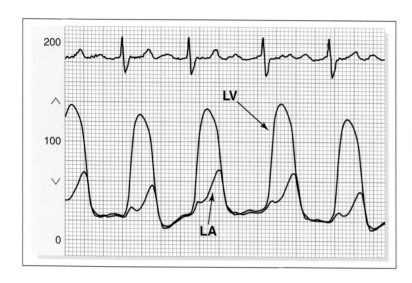

FIGURE 5-11. Simultaneous left atrial (*LA*) and left ventricular (*LV*) pressures.

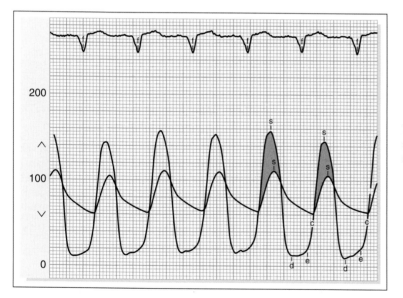

FIGURE 5-12. Simultaneous left ventricular and aortic pressures obtained in a patient with aortic stenosis demonstrating a systolic pressure gradient (*shaded*).

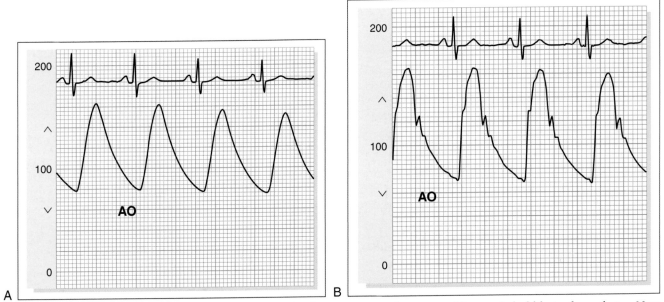

A   B

FIGURE 5-13.   *A*, Example of an overdamped aortic (AO) pressure waveform caused by an air bubble in the catheter. Note the smoothed appearance and lack of a dicrotic notch. *B*, A high-fidelity tracing is apparent after flushing.

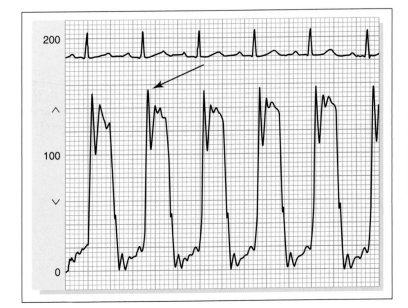

FIGURE 5-14.   Ring" artifact is common and usually caused by the presence of a small bubble located between the catheter tip and the transducer. The small bubble oscillates, causing the high-frequency, spiked artifact shown here *(arrow)*. This can usually be corrected by flushing the catheter.

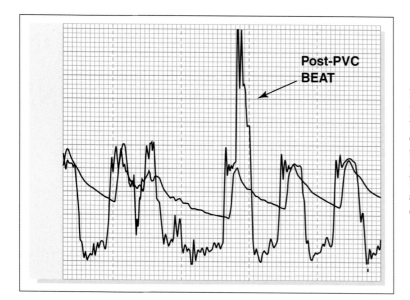

FIGURE 5-15. Catheter entrapment artifact in a patient with marked left ventricular hypertrophy undergoing catheterization to determine the presence of a left ventricular outflow tract gradient. Note that the beginning phase of ventricular systole in the postpremature ventricular contraction (post-PVC) beat appears similar to other beats but is followed by a deflection representing intramyocardial pressure caused by catheter entrapment.

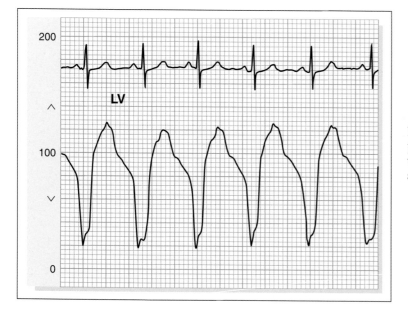

FIGURE 5-16. Hybrid waveform obtained from a pigtail catheter placed only partially within the left ventricle (*LV*). Some of the side holes of the catheter are in the aorta, causing this peculiar waveform.

CHAPTER 6

Classic Hemodynamic Waveforms in Common Pathologic Conditions

The diagnosis and management of many important cardiovascular conditions hinges on accurate collection and interpretation of hemodynamic waveforms obtained in the cardiac catheterization laboratory. Detailed descriptions of the hemodynamic findings of these conditions exceed the scope of this edition and have been described elsewhere (1). The classic hemodynamic waveforms of several cardiac conditions commonly seen in the catheterization laboratory are summarized here.

Aortic Valve Disease. Both regurgitation and stenosis of the aortic valve result in important and characteristic hemodynamic abnormalities. In both aortic regurgitation and aortic stenosis, a prominent anacrotic notch may appear on the upstroke of the aortic pressure waveform indicating flow turbulence (Fig. 6-1).

Chronic aortic regurgitation is associated with high systolic pressure and low diastolic pressure yielding a wide pulse pressure (Fig. 6-2). In severe, compensated, chronic aortic regurgitation, the early left ventricular diastolic pressure is usually normal. With the regurgitant volume, the pressure increases by end diastole and approaches the aortic diastolic pressure, a phenomenon known as *diastasis* (Fig. 6-3). With decompensation, marked increase of the left ventricular end-diastolic pressure occurs. Acute aortic regurgitation is associated with shock and pulmonary edema. Marked increase of the left ventricular end-diastolic pressure occurs, and diastasis is common. By mid or late diastole, left ventricular diastolic pressure may exceed left atrial pressure, causing preclosure of the mitral valve (Fig. 6-4).

The presence of a systolic pressure gradient across the aortic valve defines aortic stenosis, and the severity of stenosis correlates with the extent of the pressure gradient (Fig. 6-5). Quantifying the transvalvular pressure gradient is necessary for valve area calculations. Numerous methods have been used to obtain this measurement, and several of these techniques are prone to significant error (2). The ideal catheter configuration records pressure simultaneously from the left ventricle and the aorta with one catheter positioned directly above the aortic valve from a retrograde arterial approach and the other catheter placed by a transseptal approach from the femoral vein into the left ventricle toward the apex. This arrangement avoids the concern about catheter-related obstruction occurring when the valve is crossed retrograde. This method is technically more demanding and is rarely practiced unless the aortic valve cannot be crossed by a retrograde approach. The use of two separate catheters, one placed retrograde across the aortic valve into the left ventricle and a second catheter positioned from another arterial site in the ascending aorta just above the valve, provides high-quality hemodynamic data but requires two arterial punctures potentially increasing the risk for a vascular complication. Currently, the most practical and accurate method utilizes a dual-lumen pigtail catheter (or Langston catheter) allowing simultaneous pressure measurements above and below the valve from a single arterial access site.

In addition to the transvalvular pressure gradient, several additional hemodynamic abnormalities have been observed. Turbulent flow across the valve results in an anacrotic notch, and marked delay exists in the upstroke of the central aortic pressure waveform (Fig. 6-6). Pulsus alternans is a rare finding in patients with severe aortic stenosis and is usually associated with heart failure and poor left ventricular function (Fig. 6-7). In some cases of severe aortic stenosis, the profile of the catheter placed in a retrograde fashion across the aortic valve to measure left ventricular pressure contributes to obstruction. This manifests as an increase in the aortic pressure of at least 5 mm Hg when the catheter is withdrawn from the left ventricle, known as *Carabello's sign* (3) (Fig. 6-8).

Hypertrophic Obstructive Cardiomyopathy. The dynamic outflow tract obstruction characterizing hypertrophic obstructive cardiomyopathy leads to interesting hemodynamic findings. The pressure gradient between the left ventricle and aorta is due to left ventricular outflow tract obstruction from systolic anterior motion of the mitral valve. A pressure gradient may exist at rest (Fig. 6-9) or may be present only with provocation; furthermore, the resting gradient may be seen to vary spontaneously. The aortic pressure waveform has a characteristic appearance known as a "spike and dome" configuration (Fig. 6-10). This morphology differs from the aortic pressure waveform appearance when there is fixed obstruction from valvular aortic stenosis because early ejection is relatively unimpeded and obstruction develops only as ventricular systole progresses. Dynamic obstruction is also manifest by the "Brockenbrough–Braunwald sign." This sign is described as a decrease in the aortic systolic pressure and a decrease in the aortic pulse pressure seen in the beat after a premature ventricular contraction (PVC) and is due to the enhanced contractility seen in a post-PVC beat (Fig. 6-11). In patients with suspected obstruction and an absent gradient at rest, a pressure gradient may be provoked by enhancing obstruction through a decrease in preload. Measurement of the pressure gradient while having the patient perform a Valsalva maneuver is a common method of provoking a pressure gradient (Fig. 6-12).

Mitral Valve Disease. A prominent "v" wave on the pulmonary capillary wedge pressure waveform represents the classic hemodynamic finding of acute, severe mitral valve regurgitation (Fig. 6-13). A large "v" wave may sometimes be transmitted back to the pulmonary artery pressure waveform (Fig. 6-14). Note that a large "v" wave is not always evident despite severe mitral regurgitation. The presence of a "v" wave depends on the size, pressure, and compliance of the left atrium. Patients with chronic, well-compensated, severe mitral regurgitation often have normal, physiologic "v" waves on the pulmonary capillary wedge pressure tracing.

The hemodynamic hallmark of mitral stenosis is the presence of a pressure gradient at end diastole between the left atrium (or pulmonary capillary wedge pressure) and the left ventricle (Fig. 6-15). A small gradient may be present normally in early diastole. In mild mitral stenosis, the end-diastolic gradient may be only a few millimeters of mercury (mm Hg); as mitral stenosis becomes more severe, the gradient increases and may exceed 20 mm Hg in patients with severe mitral stenosis. The gradient is dependent on heart rate; higher gradients are observed with tachycardia and will decrease with longer R-R intervals (Fig. 6-16). Two additional hemodynamic findings in mitral stenosis include a prominent "a" wave on the left atrial or pulmonary capillary wedge pressure tracing (caused by a pressure increase from the presence of obstruction during atrial contraction) (Fig. 6-17) and a prominent "v" wave on the left atrial or pulmonary capillary wedge pressure tracing from left atrial filling occurring under higher left atrial pressures (and thus on a steeper part of the left atrial compliance curve) (Fig. 6-18). Pulmonary hypertension is commonly seen in both mitral valve regurgitation and stenosis with the associated hemodynamic abnormalities including increased pulmonary artery pressures, tricuspid regurgitation, and right heart failure.

Pericardial Disease. Clinical syndromes associated with pericardial disease include acute pericarditis, effusions and tamponade, and pericardial constriction. Acute pericarditis usually causes chest pain syndromes; no hemodynamic abnormalities occur unless complicated by a significant pericardial effusion. The hemodynamics of restrictive cardiomyopathy mimic pericardial disease and are often discussed concurrently.

The impact of a pericardial effusion is highly dependent on the volume of the effusion, its rate of accumulation, and the compliance of the pericardium and cardiac chambers. Thus, a wide spectrum of hemodynamic abnormalities exists in patients with pericardial effusion, ranging from completely normal to profound cardiovascular collapse and shock.

The earliest sequelae from an effusion are an increase of the right atrial and right ventricular diastolic pressures. Classically, the "y" descent on the right atrial waveform (due to the decay in pressure from atrial emptying) is attenuated (Fig. 6-19). On the other end of the spectrum, classic tamponade is manifest by an increase and equalization of the right atrial, right ventricular diastolic, pulmonary artery diastolic, and pulmonary capillary wedge pressures (Fig. 6-20). A marked reduction in cardiac output usually occurs, and a prominent pulsus paradoxus is present (Fig. 6-21). Again, based on the variables described earlier, varying degrees of hemodynamic abnormalities between these extremes may be observed.

Constrictive pericarditis creates unique and interesting hemodynamic abnormalities. A rigid pericardium limits cardiac chamber distension and increases right atrial and right ventricular and left ventricular diastolic pressures. However, unlike tamponade, which causes compression throughout the cardiac cycle, early right and left ventricular diastolic pressures are low. This leads to the characteristic hemodynamic finding of a prominent "x" and "y" descent on the right atrial waveform (Fig. 6-22), and a "square root sign" inscribed on the diastolic pressure contour of the right and left ventricular waveforms (Fig. 6-23).

Pericardial constraint also results in an increase in ventricular interdependence and a dissociation of the cardiac chambers from the changes in thoracic pressure occurring during the respiratory cycle. An increase in ventricular interdependence causes the right and left ventricular diastolic pressures to run within 1 to 2 mm Hg of each other (see Fig. 6-23). The isolation of the cardiac chambers from the pressure changes caused by respiration leads to the characteristic finding of discordance between the left and right ventricular systolic pressures (4). Normally, right and left ventricular systolic pressures are concordant during the respiratory cycle (Fig. 6-24); pericardial constriction causes discordance with the highest left ventricular systolic pressure associated with the lowest right ventricular systolic pressure and the lowest left ventricular systolic pressure associated with the highest right ventricular systolic pressure (Figs. 6-25 and 6-26).

Restrictive cardiomyopathy is a rare set of disorders with numerous causative factors and is characterized by heart failure in the presence of normal systolic function. Hemodynamic abnormalities mimic pericardial constriction. The right atrial pressure is typically markedly increased with prominent "x" and "y" descents. Right and left ventricular diastolic pressures are also increased and usually exhibit the "square root" sign. However, because the pericardium is normal, the cardiac chambers are exposed to thoracic pressure changes associated with the respiratory cycle; thus, this condition may be readily distinguished from pericardial constriction by demonstrating concordance between the right and left ventricular systolic pressures.

Congestive Heart Failure. The hemodynamic findings observed in patients with congestive heart failure caused by systolic left ventricular dysfunction are relatively nonspecific and may be seen in any condition causing left heart failure. Heart failure increases the pulmonary capillary wedge pressure and, because the right heart is in direct series, also causes passive increase of the right-sided pressures. Chronic heart failure leads to pulmonary hypertension both from reactive and fixed increases in pulmonary vascular resistance, and the sequelae of secondary tricuspid regurgitation and right heart failure.

Hemodynamic abnormalities unique to systolic dysfunction are unusual. Left ventricular end-diastolic pressure is typically increased and a prominent "a" wave may be present

(Fig. 6-27). Profound depression in left ventricular function may manifest as a triangular appearance to the left ventricular pressure waveform from the delay to reach peak systolic pressure because of diminished contractility (Fig. 6-28). Severely reduced contractile function may also cause pulsus alternans on the aortic or left ventricular pressure waveform (Fig. 6-29).

Right-Sided Cardiac Disorders. Long-standing pulmonary hypertension, regardless of the cause, ultimately leads to right ventricular hypertrophy and right-sided heart failure. Hypertrophy decreases the compliance of the right ventricle; this may be observed as a prominent "a" wave on the right ventricular pressure waveform (Fig. 6-30). Similar to left heart failure, pulsus alternans may be present on right-sided chamber pressure waveforms (i.e., right ventricle and pulmonary artery) in patients with profound right-sided heart failure (Fig. 6-31).

Tricuspid regurgitation may occur from a primary valvular disorder such as rheumatic heart disease, or may be secondary to pulmonary hypertension or right heart failure. A prominent "v" wave on the right atrial pressure waveform represents the classically described hemodynamic abnormality (Fig. 6-32). In severe cases, complete ventricularization of the right atrial waveform may occur (Fig. 6-33). Tricuspid stenosis is rare and usually caused by rheumatic heart disease. The condition is diagnosed by the presence of a diastolic pressure gradient between the right atrium and the right ventricle (Fig. 6-34).

Other right-sided conditions are due primarily to congenital heart disease, and include pulmonic stenosis and pulmonic regurgitation. Valvular pulmonic stenosis causes a systolic pressure gradient between the main pulmonary artery and the right ventricle; peripheral pulmonary stenosis causes a gradient between the right ventricle and a distal branch of the affected pulmonary artery. Severe pulmonic regurgitation is most commonly seen as a consequence of congenital heart surgery and classically appears as a wide pulse pressure or even ventricularization on the pulmonary artery waveform (Fig. 6-35).

References

1. Ragosta M: Textbook of Clinical Hemodynamics. Philadelphia, Saunders, 2008.
2. Fusman B, Faxon D, Feldman T: Hemodynamic rounds: Transvalvular pressure gradient measurement. Catheter Cardiovasc Interv 2001;53:553–561.
3. Carabello BA, Green LH, Grossman W, et al: Hemodynamic determinants of prognosis of aortic valve replacement in critical aortic stenosis and advanced congestive heart failure. Circulation 1980;62:42–48.
4. Hurrell DG, Nishimura RA, Higano ST, et al: Value of dynamic respiratory changes in left and right ventricular pressures for the diagnosis of constrictive pericarditis. Circulation 1996;93:2007–2013.

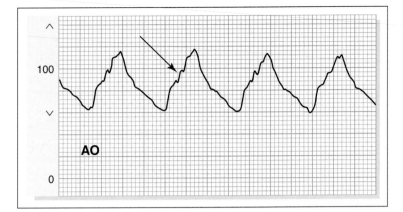

FIGURE 6-1. A prominent anacrotic "notch" or "shoulder" is shown on this central aortic (AO) waveform in a patient with severe aortic regurgitation. This finding may also be observed in patients with severe aortic stenosis and indicates turbulence during ejection.

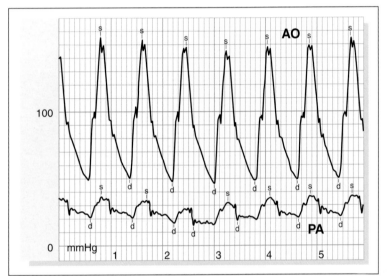

FIGURE 6-2. Severe, chronic aortic regurgitation often leads to a wide pulse pressure and systolic hypertension. AO, aorta; PA, pulmonary artery.

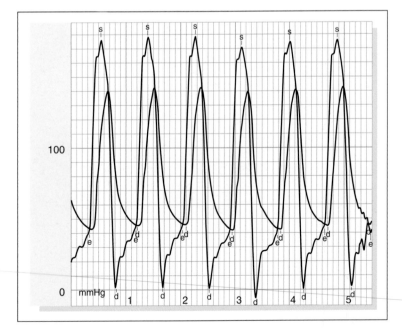

FIGURE 6-3. The phenomenon of diastasis is shown on these tracings depicting simultaneous left ventricular and femoral artery sheath pressure in a patient with severe aortic regurgitation from a degenerated bioprosthetic aortic valve. Note the rapid increase in left ventricular diastolic pressure and equalization of the left ventricular end-diastolic and arterial diastolic pressure (known as *diastasis*). There is also a systolic pressure gradient across this failing prosthetic valve.

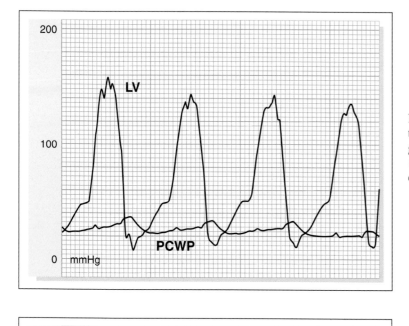

FIGURE 6-4. Example of hemodynamics obtained in a patient with severe, acute aortic regurgitation and marked increase in the left ventricular (*LV*) diastolic pressure exceeding the pulmonary capillary wedge pressure (*PCWP*).

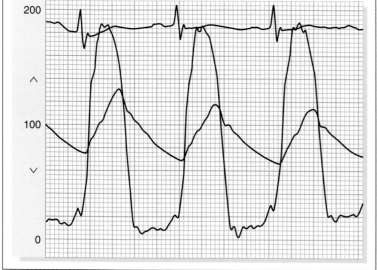

FIGURE 6-5. Simultaneous left ventricular and central aortic pressure in a patient with severe aortic stenosis. In this case, the left ventricular pressure was recorded from a catheter placed into the left ventricle by a trans-septal approach, and central aortic pressure was recorded from a catheter positioned just above the aortic valve from a retrograde approach via the femoral artery. These tracings demonstrate all of the characteristics of severe aortic stenosis including a marked delay in upstroke and the presence of a large systolic pressure gradient.

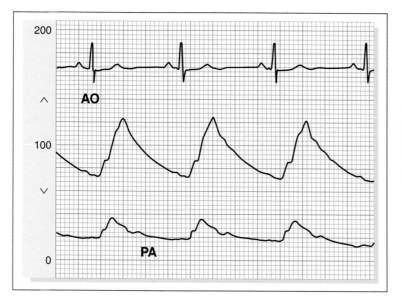

FIGURE 6-6. Example of an anacrotic notch and a marked delay in upstroke present on the aortic pressure tracing in a patient with severe aortic stenosis. AO, aorta; PA, pulmonary artery.

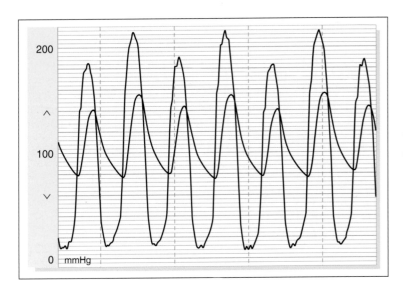

FIGURE 6-7. Pulsus alternans in a patient with severe aortic stenosis.

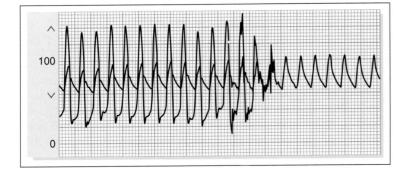

FIGURE 6-8. During pullback of a pigtail catheter from the left ventricle to the aorta, the systolic pressure in the aortic waveform increases consistent with relief of additional obstruction caused by the profile of the catheter in a patient with severe aortic stenosis (Carabello's sign).

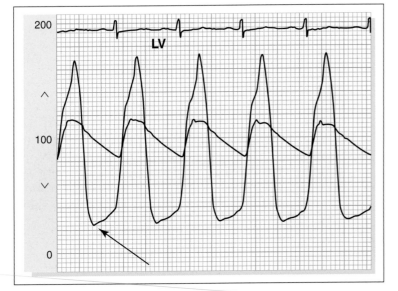

FIGURE 6-9. Simultaneous left ventricular and aortic pressure waveforms obtained in a patient with hypertrophic obstructive cardiomyopathy. There is a large pressure gradient present at rest. Note the increased, early left ventricular (*LV*) diastolic pressure consistent with diastolic dysfunction (*arrow*).

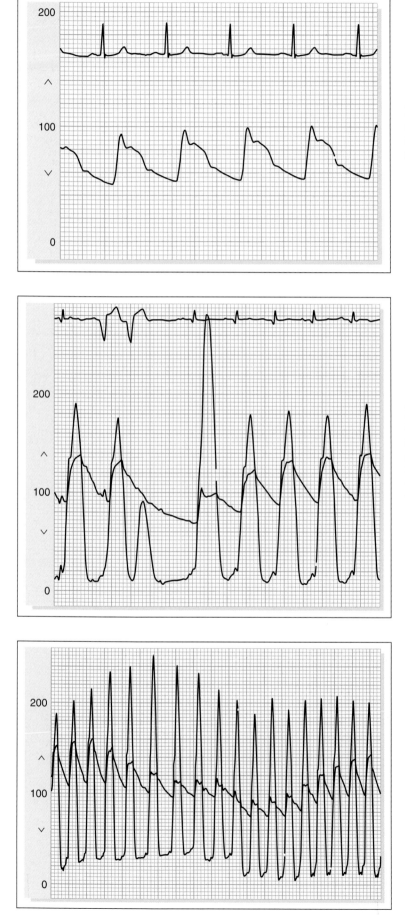

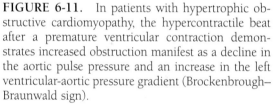

FIGURE 6-10. This aortic pressure waveform demonstrates the classic "spike-and-dome" configuration due to unobstructed early ejection followed by dynamic obstruction.

FIGURE 6-11. In patients with hypertrophic obstructive cardiomyopathy, the hypercontractile beat after a premature ventricular contraction demonstrates increased obstruction manifest as a decline in the aortic pulse pressure and an increase in the left ventricular–aortic pressure gradient (Brockenbrough–Braunwald sign).

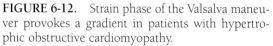

FIGURE 6-12. Strain phase of the Valsalva maneuver provokes a gradient in patients with hypertrophic obstructive cardiomyopathy.

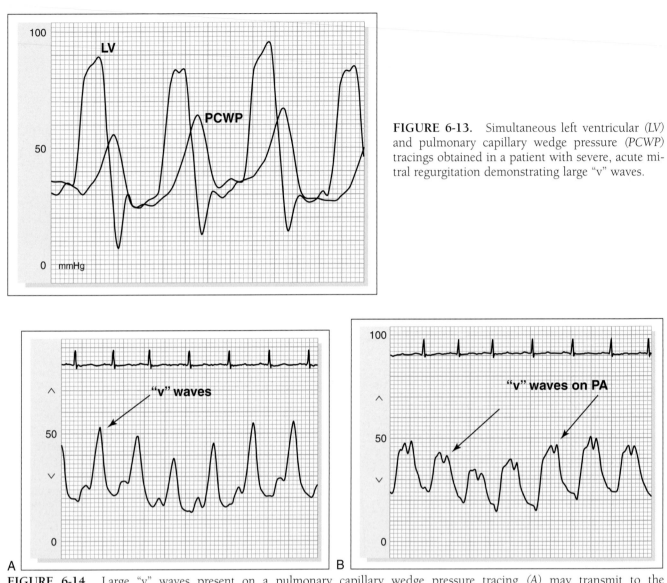

FIGURE 6-13. Simultaneous left ventricular (*LV*) and pulmonary capillary wedge pressure (*PCWP*) tracings obtained in a patient with severe, acute mitral regurgitation demonstrating large "v" waves.

FIGURE 6-14. Large "v" waves present on a pulmonary capillary wedge pressure tracing (*A*) may transmit to the pulmonary artery (*PA*) pressure tracing (*B*).

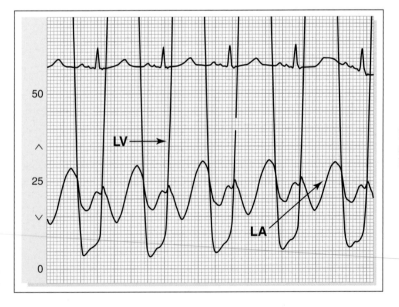

FIGURE 6-15. Mitral stenosis is characterized by a pressure gradient between the left atrium (*LA*) and left ventricle (*LV*) throughout diastole.

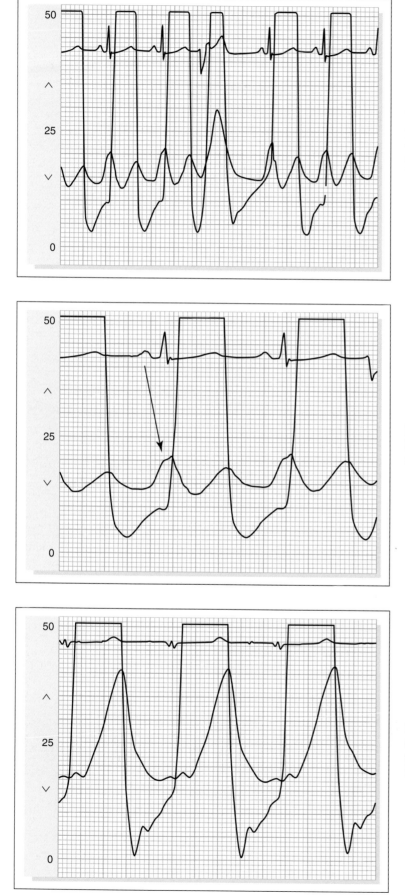
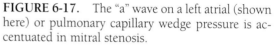

FIGURE 6-16.   Effect of a pause on the transmitral pressure gradient. Note that the gradient is largest with the shorter R-R interval and decreases with a pause.

FIGURE 6-17.   The "a" wave on a left atrial (shown here) or pulmonary capillary wedge pressure is accentuated in mitral stenosis.

FIGURE 6-18.   The "v" wave may also be markedly increased in patients with mitral stenosis. This patient with mitral stenosis has no mitral regurgitation and normal systolic function.

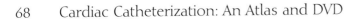

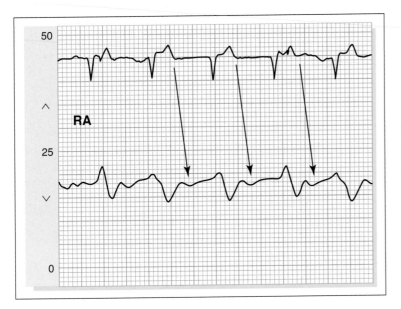

FIGURE 6-19. One of the earliest hemodynamic abnormalities in pericardial tamponade is loss of the "y" descent on the right atrial (RA) pressure waveform.

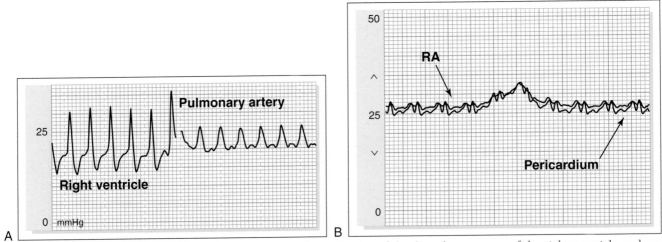

FIGURE 6-20. Classic tamponade results in increase and equalization of the diastolic pressures of the right ventricle, pulmonary artery (A), right atrium (RA), and pericardium (B).

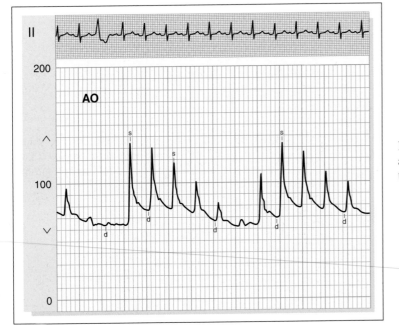

FIGURE 6-21. Marked pulsus paradox on the aortic (AO) pressure waveform in a patient with tamponade.

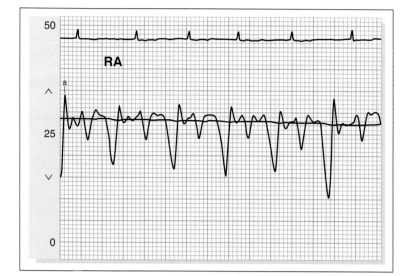

FIGURE 6-22. In pericardial constriction, the right atrial (RA) pressure is increased and the waveform is characterized by an exaggerated "y" descent.

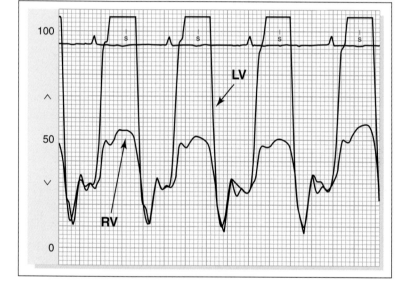

FIGURE 6-23. An additional finding in pericardial constriction is the "square root" sign and equilibration of the right (RV) and left ventricular (LV) diastolic pressures.

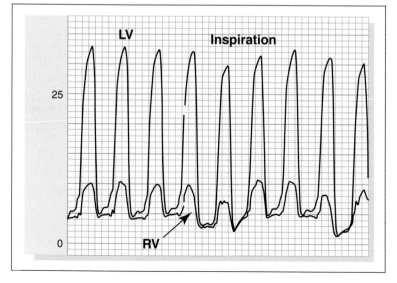

FIGURE 6-24. In patients *without* pericardial constriction (shown here), the left (LV) and right ventricular (RV) systolic pressures are concordant during the pressure changes occurring during respiration. Constriction causes discordance of the systolic pressures.

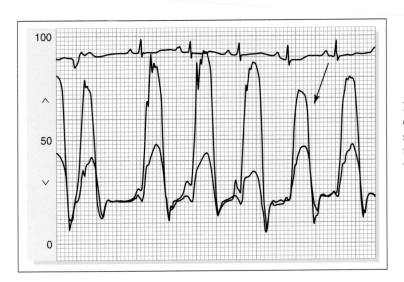

FIGURE 6-25. These tracings provide an example of discordance between the right and left ventricular systolic pressures in a patient with constriction. Note that the right ventricular systolic pressure is highest when the left ventricular systolic pressure is lowest (*arrow*).

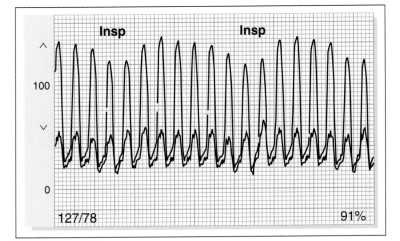

FIGURE 6-26. These tracings are another example of discordance between the right and left ventricular systolic pressures in a patient with constriction.

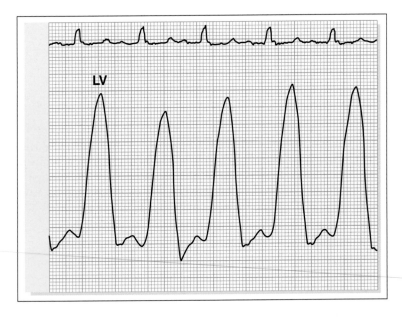

FIGURE 6-27. This left ventricular (*LV*) pressure waveform was obtained in a patient with severe left ventricular dysfunction and demonstrates a prominent "a" wave.

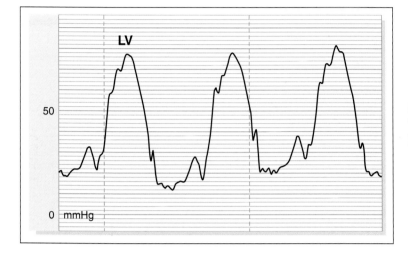

FIGURE 6-28. The left ventricular (*LV*) pressure waveform may exhibit a triangular appearance in patients with profound left ventricular dysfunction.

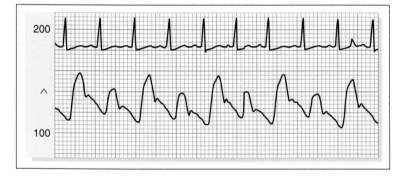

FIGURE 6-29. This aortic pressure tracing is an example of pulsus alternans, caused by severe left ventricular dysfunction.

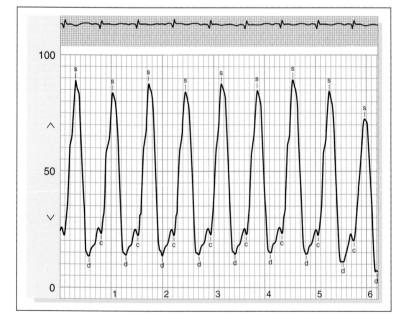

FIGURE 6-30. Patients with right ventricular hypertrophy caused by pulmonary hypertension often have prominent "a" waves on the right ventricular pressure waveform.

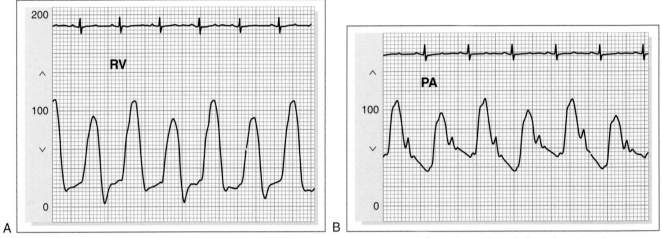

FIGURE 6-31.   Pulsus alternans may be seen on pressure waveforms obtained from the right-sided cardiac chambers in patients with right-sided heart failure. *A*, A right ventricular (*RV*) waveform depicts this finding. *B*, A pulmonary artery (*PA*) waveform demonstrates this finding.

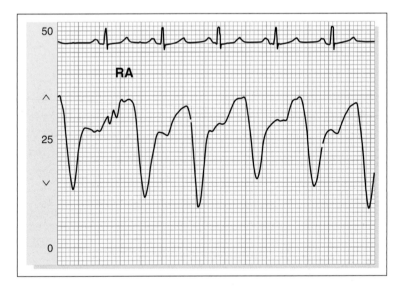

FIGURE 6-32.   Large "v" waves in the right atrial (*RA*) pressure waveform are characteristic of severe tricuspid regurgitation.

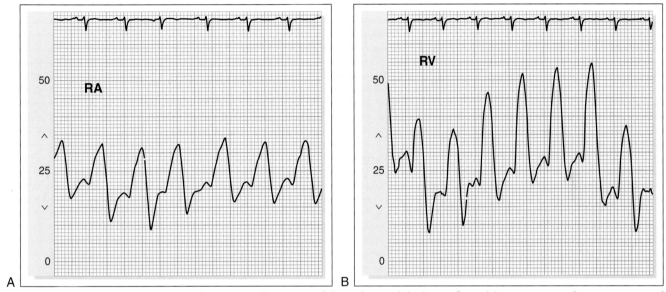

FIGURE 6-33. There may be complete ventricularization of the right atrial (*RA*) waveform (*A*) in patients with severe tricuspid regurgitation. *B*, Same patient's right ventricular (*RV*) pressure.

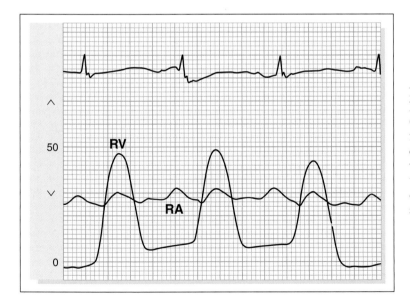

FIGURE 6-34. This pressure waveform was collected from a 19-year-old patient with a mechanical (tilting disc) tricuspid valve presenting with severe right-sided heart failure and thrombosis of the mechanical valve. The right ventricular (*RV*) pressure waveform was obtained via right ventricular puncture. The right atrial (*RA*) pressure is markedly increased with a prominent "a" wave and a large diastolic pressure gradient.

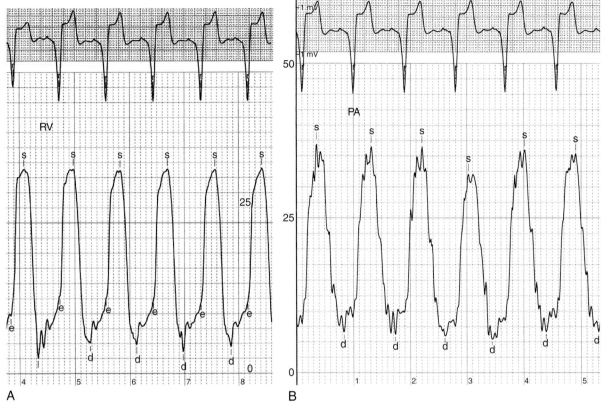

A

B

FIGURE 6-35.   These tracings were obtained from a patient with severe pulmonic insufficiency after surgical correction of tetralogy of Fallot. A, Right ventricular (RV) pressure. B, Pulmonary artery (PA) pressure. Note the wide pulse pressure on the pulmonary artery tracing with equilibration of diastolic pressures.

LEFT VENTRICULOGRAPHY

Left ventriculography is an important component of a routine left heart catheterization used to quantify left ventricular function and to identify the presence and severity of mitral valve regurgitation. Left ventriculography can also reveal the presence of left ventricular hypertrophy and demonstrate other abnormalities such as ventricular septal defects, left ventricular thrombus, and ventricular aneurysms. Ventriculography can also provide information regarding right ventricular size, the presence of coronary anomalies, and diseases of the aorta.

Left ventriculography adds little additional risk to a cardiac catheterization and should be routinely performed in all diagnostic left heart catheterizations unless there is a specific reason not to. Left ventriculography is commonly deferred in patients with renal insufficiency in whom it is desirable to limit the volume of contrast, and in patients with marked increases of pulmonary capillary wedge pressure or left ventricular end-diastolic pressure who may not tolerate the hemodynamic effects of a contrast bolus. It is advisable to avoid ventriculography in the presence of a mobile left ventricular thrombus seen on echocardiography or in cases of active aortic valve endocarditis. Although patients with aortic valve stenosis can safely undergo ventriculography, great care should be taken in patients with severe aortic stenosis and tenuous hemodynamics because the vasodilatory effects of contrast may cause hypotension and hemodynamic collapse.

Power Injector. Several angiographic procedures performed in the cardiac catheterization laboratory require the delivery of large volumes of radiocontrast agent delivered at high flow rates under relatively high pressures not practical by hand injection. These include left or right ventriculography, aortography, and pulmonary angiography. The *power injector,* a long-standing fixture of cardiac catheterization laboratories, serves this purpose. Understanding the proper use of this important tool is necessary to attain the highest quality diagnostic images during these angiographic procedures.

Power injectors are available in various styles and by numerous manufacturers. Four variables can be adjusted by the operator and include: (a) the volume of contrast in milliliters; (b) the rate of contrast injection in milliliters per second; (c) the time, in seconds, until peak injection rate occurs or "rate of rise"; and (d) the maximum pressure used for injection in pounds per square inch (psi). The volume of contrast depends on the study; right or left ventriculography often requires 30 to 40 mL, arch aortography requires 60 mL, abdominal aortography with lower extremity runoff requires 80 to 120 mL. The rate of contrast injection also varies depending on the study. The greatest flow rates are used in the ascending aorta (20–30 mL/sec); ventriculography uses 12 to 15 mL/sec, and lower extremity runoff needs only 8 to 10 mL/sec. The rate of rise is adjusted for ventriculograms to prevent ectopy. This is typically set at 0.8 second for these studies, which means that it requires 0.8 second until the desired flow rate is actually achieved. This adjustment is not necessary for aortography (rate of rise set at 0). The maximum pressure programmed by the operator defines the highest pressure that will be used to deliver the contrast at the desired flow rate; this is usually set at 600 psi. If substantial resistance occurs, the power injector will not exceed this pressure limit; thus, the flow rate will be lower than that requested. For this reason, when high flow rates are required, the maximum pressure should be adjusted to the maximum pressure tolerated by the catheter chosen (usually 1000–1200 psi). If this still provides inadequate flow rates, a larger caliber catheter is needed.

Performance of Left Ventriculography. Left ventriculography is typically accomplished using a pigtail catheter with multiple side holes. The aortic valve is crossed as described in Chapter 4. On entering the left ventricle, the operator should be attentive to the cardiac rhythm because significant ectopy may result from the pigtail catheter in the ventricle; gentle repositioning of the catheter usually restores a stable rhythm. The optimal catheter position is in the midcavity of the left ventricle in the left ventricular inflow tract just in front of the mitral valve. Review of the pressure waveform and absence of the appearance of a hybrid left ventricular pressure tracing (Fig. 7-1) ensures that all the holes of the pigtail catheter are within the left ventricle. Ventriculography should not be performed until the rhythm is stable and the catheter position is optimal.

Contrast is injected into the left ventricle with a power injector. When connecting the catheter to the power injection, great care should be taken to be sure there are no air bubbles in the catheter or in the column of contrast in the power injector. Typically, a test injection using 5 mL of contrast confirms that the catheter position is appropriate and can also help estimate the volume of contrast required. On average, 35 to 40 mL of contrast injected at a flow rate of 12 to 14 mL/sec provides excellent opacification of the left ventricle. A rate of rise of 0.8 second is used to help reduce the chance of ventricular ectopy. Inadequate opacification prevents identification of wall motion abnormalities, makes quantification of mitral regurgitation unreliable, and obscures subtle abnormalities such as the presence of a left ventricular thrombus or a ventricular pseudoaneurysm. Larger volumes (45–55 mL) of contrast may be needed when ventricular enlargement or chronic mitral regurgitation with atrial enlargement is present.

When ventriculography is performed in a biplane laboratory, the typical angles are 30 degrees right anterior oblique (RAO) and 60 degrees left anterior oblique (LAO). The RAO projection is preferred when only a single imaging plane is available. If mitral regurgitation is suspected, additional RAO angulation may be required to remove the overlap of the aorta and left atrium. This can be determined during the test injection by comparing the catheter position in the descending aorta with the position of the mitral annulus. If necessary, additional RAO angulation will prevent the left atrium from overlapping the descending aorta providing a clear view of the extent of mitral regurgitation.

An example of a high-quality left ventriculogram is shown in Videos 7-1 and 7-2. Note the catheter position and the dense opacification of the left ventricle with the presence of a stable rhythm during injection. The pigtail catheter is often improperly positioned leading to poor-quality ventriculograms. If the catheter is positioned in the left ventricular apex (Video 7-3), power injection predictably causes substantial ectopy and a difficult-to-interpret ventriculogram. Even properly positioned catheters may cause significant ectopy and artifactual mitral regurgitation (Video 7-4). Use of an inadequate volume of contrast incompletely opacifies the left ventricle, obscuring wall motion abnormalities and the degree of mitral regurgitation, and preventing the identification of subtle findings (Video 7-5). These errors can be easily avoided by the use of careful technique.

Determination of Left Ventricular Function. Estimation of left ventricular systolic function and identification of regional myocardial dysfunction are the most common indications for left ventriculography. Global ventricular systolic function is typically described by calculation of the ejection fraction. Using computer-assisted algorithms applied to a high-quality ventriculogram, the left ventricular end-systolic and end-diastolic contours are traced (Fig, 7-2). Diastolic and systolic areas can be determined and the corresponding ventricular volumes calculated based on assumptions regarding the geometry of the heart. The left ventricular ejection fraction (LVEF) can be easily calculated by the following formula:

$$LVEF = 1 - (\text{end-systolic volume/end-diastolic volume})$$

Determination of regional left ventricular function is an important part of the assessment of patients with coronary artery disease. Typically, the ventricle is divided into several segments loosely based on the usual vascular distribution of the coronary arteries. A commonly used system divides the ventricle into 5 segments in each of the RAO and LAO views yielding 10 segments for analysis if biplane ventriculography is performed (Fig. 7-3). Segmental function is described semiquantitatively. Each segment is classified as "normal" if it contracts well, "hypokinetic" if there is reduced or minimal contraction, "akinetic" if there is no contraction of the segment, or "dyskinetic" if the segment moves outward during systole. The ventriculographic grading of wall motion is a subjective interpretation with some variance between observers.

The usual relation between the various regional myocardial segments and the major coronary arteries is shown in Table 7-1. These relations are subject to wide variation depending on unique aspects of an individual's coronary anatomy. For example, in some patients, the apex of the heart is supplied by the right coronary artery as a continuation of the posterior descending artery and not by the left anterior descending artery (Video 7-6). In the presence of a large, dominant circumflex, the inferior as well as the lateral and posterior walls of the heart are supplied by this vessel and not by the right coronary artery. Right coronary arteries exhibit great variation in the size of the posterolateral and posterior descending arteries relative to the branches of the circumflex; thus, it may be difficult to distinguish circumflex infarctions from right coronary events based solely on ventriculography. Many cardiac catheterization laboratories perform ventriculography in only the RAO view and may potentially miss wall motion abnormalities involving the circumflex artery because the posterior walls are seen only on LAO views. Typical examples of regional wall motion abnormalities involving commonly observed coronary artery distributions are provided in Videos 7-7 through 7-11.

Determination of Presence and Extent of Mitral Regurgitation. Ventriculography offers the ability to diagnose and quantify the degree of mitral valve regurgitation. Again, it is imperative to obtain a high-quality ventriculogram because inadequate contrast volume or improper catheter position causes error in the estimation of the severity of mitral regurgitation, and excessive ectopy creates artifactual regurgitation.

Mitral regurgitation is graded using a semiquantitative scale (Table 7-2). Although this scale is helpful, it is important to realize that the operator may underestimate the severity of mitral regurgitation when there is marked left atrial enlargement because there may not be complete or dense opacification of the left atrium despite the presence of severe regurgitation. In addition, the operator should beware of artifactual mitral regurgitation caused by excessive ventricular ectopy (see Video 7-4) or improper catheter position. Examples of varying grades (1+ to 4+) of mitral regurgitation are shown in Videos 7-12 through 7-15, and examples of various conditions associated with mitral regurgitation are shown in Videos 7-16 through 7-20.

Table 7-1. Relation between Myocardial Segments Seen on Left Ventriculography and Coronary Artery Vascular Territories

CORONARY ARTERY	SEGMENTS
Left anterior descending	Anterolateral Apical Septal
Diagonal branches	Anterolateral
Ramus intermedius	Anterolateral Superolateral
Left circumflex (dominant right coronary artery)	Posterolateral Superolateral
Dominant right coronary artery	Posterobasal Diaphragmatic Inferolateral

Table 7-2.	Semiquantitative Scale for Assessing the Severity of Mitral Regurgitation	
DEGREE	**VENTRICULOGRAPHIC CRITERIA**	
1+	Faint opacification of the left atrium with clearing of contrast during each beat	
2+	Opacification of the atrium that does not clear but is not as dense as the left ventricle	
3+	Opacification of the atrium with the same density as the ventricle	
4+	Immediate, dense opacification of the atrium with filling of the pulmonary veins	

Diagnosis of Other Conditions by Left Ventriculography. Additional pathologic conditions can be demonstrated by left ventriculography. Ventriculography provides an image of the ventricular lumen, and although it does not provide direct information regarding the presence of left ventricular hypertrophy, enlargement of the papillary muscles may be readily apparent on ventriculography (Video 7-21). Hypertrophic cardiomyopathy is a condition with excessive hypertrophy and a characteristic ventriculogram. In patients with hypertrophic cardiomyopathy, cavity obliteration is commonly seen together with small ventricular end-systolic volumes (Video 7-22). When associated ventricular outflow tract obstruction also is present, systolic anterior motion of the mitral valve (the underlying cause of obstruction) results in severe degrees of mitral regurgitation (Video 7-23). The ventriculogram in the apical variant of hypertrophic cardiomyopathy typically appears with a "spade"-shaped contour (Videos 7-24 and 7-25).

Filling defects appearing within the left ventricle on ventriculography usually represent a mural thrombus and occur in the setting of recent acute infarction. Most ventricular thrombi are apical in location and associated with anteroapical infarction (Videos 7-26 and 7-27). Other conditions that cause a filling defect in the left ventricle are rare and include hypertrophied papillary muscles, cardiac tumor, or a vegetation from endocarditis.

Left ventriculography is an excellent method of demonstrating both congenital and acquired ventricular septal defects (Videos 7-28 and 7-29). The LAO cranial or "hepatoclavicular" view (60 degrees LAO and 20 degrees cranial) provides an excellent view of the full extent of the ventricular septum with minimal foreshortening. Ventriculography in the RAO projection obscures the location of the septal defect because the right ventricle overlies the septum in this view. In the RAO view, a ventricular septal defect manifests by the presence of a left-to-right shunt with the appearance of contrast in the pulmonary artery and outflow tract (Video 7-30).

Left ventricular aneurysms are a potential complication of myocardial infarction. On ventriculography, a true left ventricular aneurysm is characterized by a diastolic deformity and either akinesis or dyskinesis of the affected segment (Videos 7-31 to 7-33). The mouth of the aneurysm is typically broad based. A ventricular pseudoaneurysm is a rare complication of infarction representing a contained free-wall rupture. This potentially lethal complication may be asymptomatic and is often clinically unsuspected. Frequently, this condition is fortuitously diagnosed by a routine echocardiogram or left ventriculogram performed for assessment of ventricular function after myocardial infarction. Classically, the neck of this aneurysm is narrow and emanates from an akinetic or hypokinetic area.

True ventricular aneurysms consist of nonviable myocardium and do not improve function. However, a recently described yet poorly understood entity known as *apical ballooning syndrome* is a condition in which there is transient, severe left ventricular dysfunction in the absence of infarction or coronary artery disease. The left ventricle often appears aneurysmal, and the condition predominantly affects the apex of the heart (Video 7-34). This syndrome is often precipitated by intense emotional stress and is also known as "takotsubo" heart for the resemblance of the left ventricle to the Japanese octopus trap.

A rare finding appearing similar to an aneurysm is a left ventricular diverticulum. This congenital condition most often affects the apex and is associated with other congenital abnormalities but may rarely be noted incidentally on ventriculography as an isolated abnormality at other locations (Video 7-35).

Enlargement of the right ventricle can be indirectly assessed by left ventriculography. Right ventricular enlargement is often due to severe pulmonary hypertension or large atrial septal defects, and causes flattening of the interventricular septum and shifting of the septum to the left readily apparent on the LAO left ventriculogram (Video 7-36).

Finally, ventriculography provides details regarding the aortic valve and the proximal segment of the aorta. Congenitally bicuspid aortic valves may be appreciated by the characteristic "doming" appearance of the valve (Video 7-37). Abnormalities of the proximal aorta (such as aortic aneurysms or dissection) may be imaged during ventriculography (Video 7-38). In addition, close scrutiny of the ventriculogram may assist the operator in finding anomalous coronary arteries or difficult-to-engage saphenous vein grafts.

References

1. Walton-Shirley M, Smith SM, Talley JD: Left ventricular diverticulum: case report and review of the literature. Cathet Cardiovasc Diagn 1992;26:31–33.
2. Prasad A, Lerman A, Rihal CS. Apical ballooning syndrome (Tako-Tsubo or stress cardiomyopathy): a mimic of acute myocardial infarction. Am Heart J 2008;155:408–417.

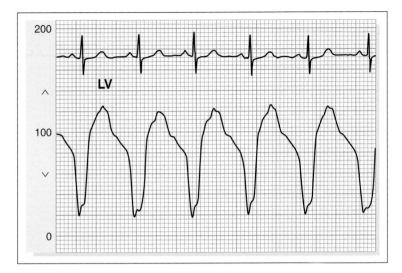

FIGURE 7-1. Tracing indicates that the pigtail catheter is not entirely within the left ventricular (LV) chamber. The more proximal side holes are within the aorta resulting in the appearance of a "hybrid" waveform, that is, between an aortic pressure waveform and left ventricular pressure waveform. If a ventriculogram is performed with the catheter in this position, the ventricular chamber will be incompletely opacified because some of the contrast will be injected into the aorta yielding a poor-quality ventriculogram.

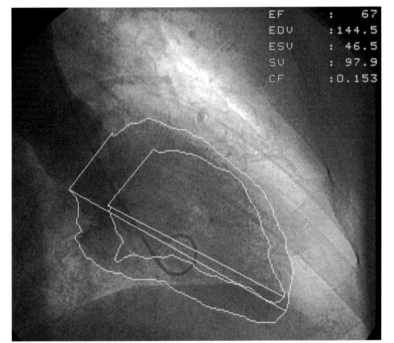

FIGURE 7-2. Example of the method used to calculate ejection fraction. End-systolic and end-diastolic contours are traced and the areas of each calculated. The following formula provides the ejection fraction, which in this case, was calculated as 67%: left ventricular ejection fraction (LVEF) = 1 − (end-systolic volume/end-diastolic volume).

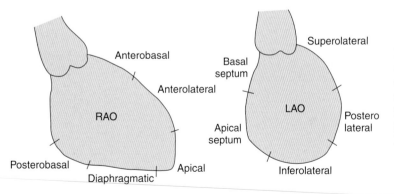

FIGURE 7-3. Regional function is described by dividing the heart into the myocardial segments shown here. Each segment can be graded as showing normal wall motion, hypokinesis (reduced systolic function), akinesis (no systolic function), or dyskinesis (systolic bulging). LAO, left anterior oblique; RAO, right anterior oblique.

AORTOGRAPHY

Angiography of the major segments of the aorta (ascending, arch, descending, and abdominal aorta) is commonly performed in the cardiac catheterization laboratory. Common indications for ascending aorta and arch aortography include the diagnosis and quantification of the extent of aortic regurgitation, diagnosis of diseases of the aorta such as thoracic aortic aneurysms and proximal aortic dissection, and evaluation of congenital defects such as coarctation of the aorta and patent ductus arteriosus. Arch aortography is also used to evaluate atherosclerotic disease at the origin of the great vessels (subclavian, carotid, or vertebral arteries). Ascending and arch aortography is sometimes performed to assist the operator in finding coronary arteries or saphenous vein grafts difficult to engage selectively. In the cardiac catheterization laboratory, abdominal aortography is often performed to diagnose renal artery stenosis or to evaluate the iliac arteries and descending aorta for peripheral arterial disease, aneurysms, or vessel tortuosity.

Ascending Aorta and Arch Aortography. Performance of this procedure requires careful attention to both catheter position and injection technique. A 6 French (Fr) pigtail catheter is positioned above the aortic valve at the level of the sinotubular junction (Fig. 8-1). If the catheter is positioned too low and sits directly on top of the aortic valve, the catheter may prolapse into the ventricle during injection, resulting in an inadequate aortogram and making it impossible to estimate the degree of aortic regurgitation. Positioning the pigtail catheter too high in the aorta does not allow complete opacification of the root of the aorta or the sinuses of Valsalva, obscuring important details of those segments of the aorta and not allowing for an accurate estimation of the degree of aortic regurgitation.

Obtaining a diagnostic quality study requires dense opacification of the aorta. This entails the injection of a relatively large volume of contrast at rapid rates to overcome the high flow rates in the large-caliber proximal aorta. Reliable studies can be achieved with 6 Fr pigtail catheters using 60 mL of contrast injected with a power injector at a rate of 30 mL/sec allowing no more than 1000 pounds per square inch (psi) injection pressure. Catheters smaller than 6 Fr do not allow for flow rates rapid enough for dense opacification. The optimal angiographic view depends on the indication for the aortogram; a 30-degree right anterior oblique view is ideal for the determination of the degree of aortic regurgitation; a 40- to 60-degree left anterior oblique view is an excellent view for identification of the origin of the coronary arteries or vein grafts and for demonstrating the extent of an aortic dissection or aneurysm. A more shallow (20–30 degrees) left anterior oblique view displays the origin of the great vessels from the arch of the aorta (Figs. 8-2 and 8-3), and a left lateral projection (90 degrees) is most useful for demonstrating a patent ductus arteriosus (Fig. 8-4).

Aortography in Aortic Valve Regurgitation. Common causes of valvular aortic regurgitation are listed in Table 8-1. Aortography provides an estimation of the degree of aortic regurgitation described by a semiquantitative scale. No contrast appears in the left ventricle when aortography is performed in the presence of a normal aortic valve. In the presence of

Table 8-1.	Causes of Aortic Regurgitation
Aortoannular ectasia
Congenital bicuspid aortic valve
Rheumatic heart disease
Endocarditis
Aortic aneurysm
Aortic dissection
Marfan syndrome
Subaortic stenosis due to membrane
Ventricular septal defect with prolapsing cusp
Ankylosing spondylitis
Rheumatoid arthritis
Syphilis
Ehlers–Danlos syndrome

mild aortic regurgitation (1+), a small amount of contrast appears in the left ventricle during diastole but clears out of the left ventricle during each systole and never completely fills the left ventricular chamber (Video 8-1). Mild-to-moderate aortic regurgitation (2+) results in faint opacification of the entire left ventricle during diastole, and the contrast remains during systole but never appears as dense as the contrast in the aorta (Video 8-2). The left ventricle progressively opacifies and appears as dense as the aorta in cases of moderately severe aortic regurgitation (3+) (Video 8-3), and severe aortic regurgitation (4+) causes complete and dense opacification of the left ventricle during the first diastole with the left ventricle becoming more densely opacified than the aorta (Video 8-4).

Aortography in Diseases of the Aorta. Aneurysms commonly involve the thoracic aorta and are readily apparent by aortography. The majority of aneurysms affect the aortic root (sinuses of Valsalva), the ascending aorta, and the descending aorta. Aneurysms of the aortic arch alone are unusual. Cystic medial necrosis represents the underlying pathology responsible for most thoracic aneurysms. Conditions associated with aneurysmal disease of the thoracic aorta are listed in Table 8-2.

Defining an aneurysm based on some arbitrary absolute dimension is problematic because the diameter of the ascending aorta varies depending on the size and sex of an individual. The ascending aorta of a normal-sized adult measures approximately 2.5 to 3.0 cm, tapering as it extends around the aortic arch to about 2.0 cm in the thoracic portion of the descending aorta. In general, ascending aortic diameters in excess of 4.0 cm are abnormal and usually represent aneurysmal disease. Although many imaging methods can be used to define thoracic aneurysms, aortography is particularly helpful in defining the maximum diameter of the

Table 8-2.	Conditions Associated with Thoracic Aortic Aneurysm
Hypertension
Congenital bicuspid aortic valve
Marfan syndrome
Ehlers–Danlos syndrome
Familial aneurysm syndromes
Turner syndrome
Atherosclerosis
Arteritis
Trauma (pseudoaneurysms)
Healed dissection

aorta, the longitudinal extent of the aneurysm, and whether associated aortic valve regurgitation or encroachment is on the great vessels. The degree of aortic valve regurgitation is particularly important in cases of large thoracic aneurysms to help determine whether the valve can be spared or will need to be replaced at the time of aneurysm repair.

Most thoracic aneurysms involve the ascending aorta and are fusiform in shape (Fig. 8-5); some are saccular. Atherosclerosis usually causes aneurysms distal to the left subclavian artery in the descending thoracic aorta. Marfan syndrome causes progressive aortic root enlargement beginning with marked dilatation of the aortic root resulting in a characteristic "cobrahead" deformity (Fig. 8-6).

Aortic dissections are also readily apparent on aortography. Patients under evaluation for suspected acute thoracic aortic dissection more often undergo imaging modalities such as computed tomography or transesophageal echocardiography to promptly and noninvasively confirm the diagnosis rather than aortography with the potential for delay in diagnosis and the associated risk of an invasive procedure. Nevertheless, aortography plays an important role in this condition. Typically, in the cardiac catheterization laboratory, suspicion for an aortic dissection may arise when a patient with risk factors for aortic dissection and ongoing chest pain initially attributed to an acute coronary syndrome is found instead to have no significant coronary obstruction. Aortography is often pursued at this junction to establish the diagnosis. Alternatively, the operator may identify the condition surreptitiously, either by noting a false lumen in the aorta on ventriculography or by observing suspicious behavior of the guide wire or catheter suggesting the presence of a false lumen.

In the cardiac catheterization laboratory, aortography both diagnoses and defines the extent of the dissection. The diagnosis is confirmed when a dissection flap is visualized, usually appearing as a linear filling defect with random motion within the lumen of the aorta (Fig. 8-7). Contrast may be retained behind the dissection flap in the false lumen or may quickly wash out if the false lumen freely communicates with the true lumen. The dissection flap may be small and a relatively subtle finding or may be extensive. Aortic dissections are usually classified by the DeBakey system. Type I dissections involve solely the ascending aorta, type II involve both the ascending and descending aorta, and type III affect only the descending aorta. If there is involvement of the aortic arch, it is important to determine the presence of associated aortic regurgitation and whether there is involvement of the great vessels. Examples of aortography in patients with varieties of thoracic aortic aneurysm and other aortic pathology are shown in Videos 8-5 through 8-11.

Abdominal Aortography. The numerous branches of the abdominal aorta can be easily demonstrated by aortography; however, most cardiologists use this technique primarily as a method to diagnose renal artery stenosis or to define pathologic conditions of the distal aorta and the iliac arteries. In such cases, a conventional pigtail catheter is positioned just above the renal arteries. Some operators utilize pigtail catheters embedded with radiopaque markers at 1-cm intervals to allow for precise measurements of vessel diameter and lesion length. Because there is great variability in the origin of the renal arteries, a small hand injection of 3 to 5 mL of contrast can help to optimally position the catheter. The T12-L1 vertebral interspace serves as an appropriate initial catheter position. Care should be taken to avoid placing the catheter too high above the renal arteries because this will result in opacification of the superior mesenteric artery potentially obscuring the origin of the renal artery and diminishing the quality of the study. After positioning the catheter at the proper location in the aorta, 25 to 40 mL of contrast is injected using the power injector at rates of 12 to 20 mL/sec at 1000 psi. Less contrast can be used if digital subtraction techniques are available. Selection of a large field of view (10–12 inches) allows visualization of a complete nephrogram resulting from renal filtration of contrast assisting in estimation of kidney size, as well as identification of accessory renal arteries, present in approximately 20% of kidneys (1). The anteroposterior (AP) projection is frequently used; however, many operators use a shallow (10–20 degree) left anterior oblique angulation to allow better visualization of the ostium of the left renal artery. Examples of abdominal aortograms used to diagnose renal artery stenosis are shown in Figures 8-8 and 8-9 and in Videos 8-12 through 8-14.

Abdominal aortography is also an excellent method of diagnosing obstructive atherosclerotic disease of the iliac arteries, identifying distal aortic or iliac artery aneurysms, and determining the presence of severe iliac tortuosity that may lead to difficulty in performing cardiac catheterization procedures from the femoral artery or prevent placement of cardiac support devices such as an intra-aortic balloon pump. When the primary focus of the study is to image the iliac arteries and distal aorta, the pigtail catheter should be positioned just above the iliac bifurcation. Typically, 25 to 30 mL of contrast injected by the power injector at 12 to 15 mL/sec results in excellent opacification. Digital subtraction techniques are not mandatory but allow lower doses of contrast and improve image quality. An AP projection with a wide field of view (15 inches) allows imaging from the distal aorta to the common femoral artery (Fig. 8-10). Additional, 30-degree right and left anterior oblique views (known as *pelvic oblique views*) are necessary to image the bifurcation of the common iliac artery into the external and internal iliac arteries, and the bifurcation of the common femoral into the superficial and profunda femoral arteries without overlap (Fig. 8-11). Examples of abdominal aortography to evaluate the iliac vessels are shown in Videos 8-15 and 8-16.

References

1. Desberg AL, Paushter DM, Lammert GK, et al: Renal artery stenosis: Evaluation with color Doppler flow imaging. Radiology 1990;177:749–753.
2. Layton KF, Kallmes DF, Cloft HJ, et al: Bovine aortic arch variant in humans: Clarification of a common misnomer. Am J Neuroradiol 2006;27:1541–1542.

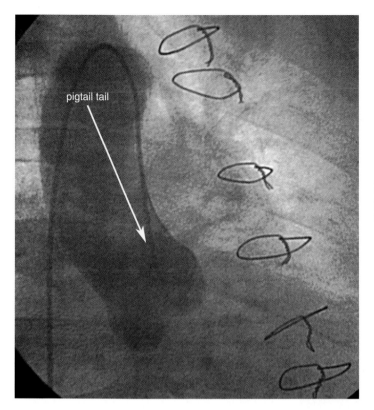

FIGURE 8-1. Proper position of pigtail catheter in the proximal aorta for performance of aortography of the aortic root.

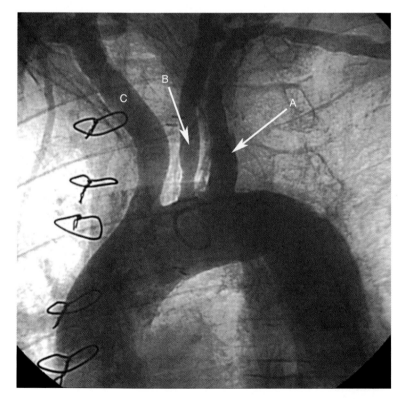

FIGURE 8-2. Aortography performed in the 20-degree left anterior oblique orientation showing the arch of the aorta and the origin of the left subclavian artery (A), the left common carotid (B), and the innominate artery (C) from the aorta.

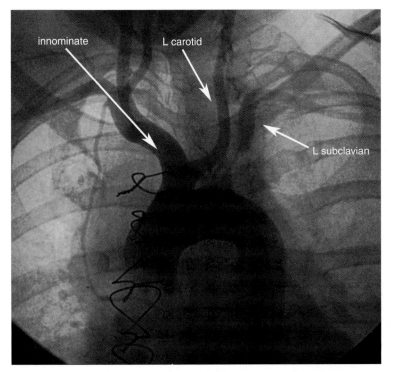

innominate

L carotid

L subclavian

FIGURE 8-3. Aortography performed in the 20-degree left anterior oblique orientation in a patient with an arch anomaly. The left carotid artery originates from the innominate instead of directly from the aortic arch. This anomaly is sometimes called a *bovine arch* (z). Severe stenosis also exists in the left subclavian artery.

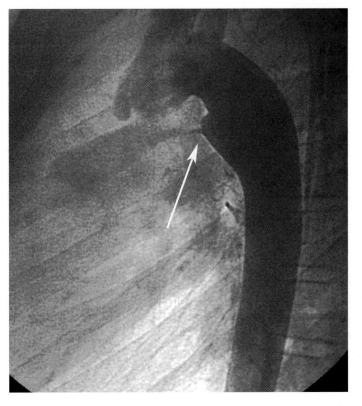

FIGURE 8-4. Aortography performed in the left lateral projection demonstrating a small patent ductus arteriosus (*arrow*).

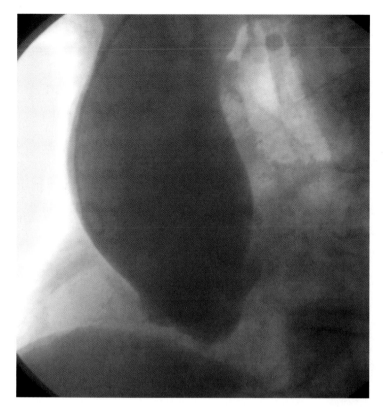

FIGURE 8-5. This aortogram demonstrates a large fusiform aneurysm of the ascending aorta. No associated aortic regurgitation was present.

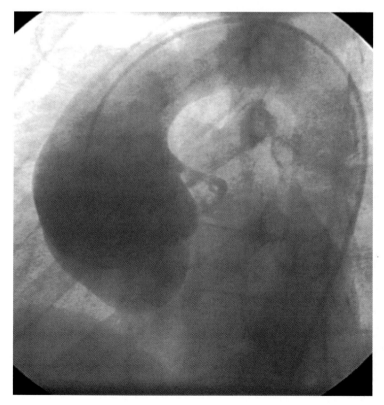

FIGURE 8-6. Characteristic appearance of an aortogram in a patient with Marfan syndrome and aneurysm of the aorta at the level of the sinuses of Valsalva showing a "cobra-head" deformity.

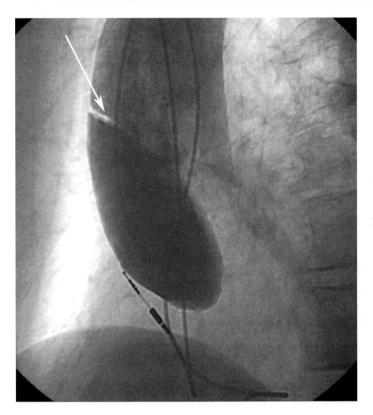

FIGURE 8-7. This left anterior oblique aortogram demonstrates aortic dissection involving the ascending aorta. A prominent dissection flap (*arrow*) with a false lumen below it is shown.

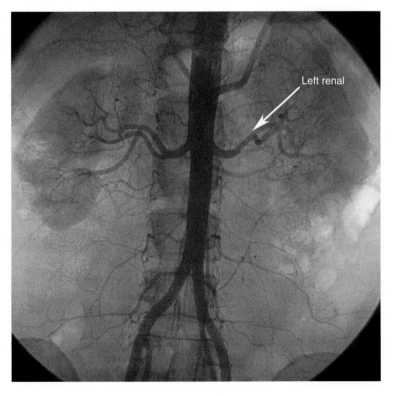

Left renal

FIGURE 8-8. Abdominal aortography performed in the anteroposterior projection demonstrating normal renal arteries.

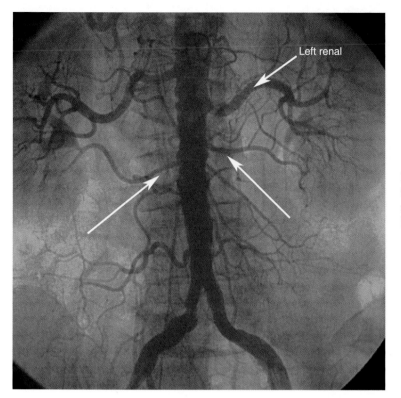

FIGURE 8-9. Abdominal aortography performed in the anteroposterior projection. An accessory renal artery can be seen supplying the lower pole of each kidney (*arrows*).

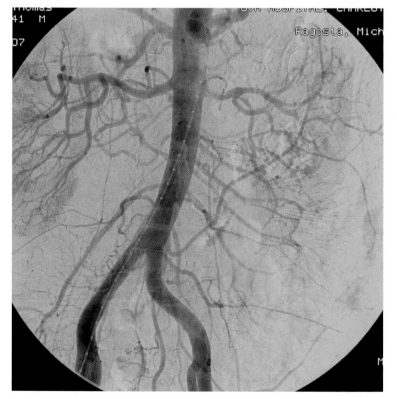

FIGURE 8-10. Example of digital subtraction angiography of the distal aorta with 10 degrees of left anterior oblique angulation. This study demonstrates normal renal arteries and a normal distal aorta and common iliac arteries.

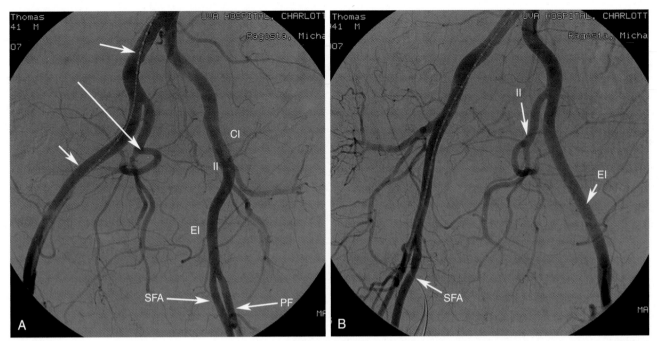

FIGURE 8-11.   Examples of digital subtraction angiography of the iliac vessels using oblique angulation to demonstrate the origin of the branches of the iliac and femoral vessels. *A,* Thirty degrees of left anterior oblique angulation is provided and clearly demonstrates the bifurcation of the right common iliac *(CI)* into the external iliac *(EI)* and internal iliac *(II)* branches. This same view demonstrates the bifurcation of the left common femoral artery into the left superficial femoral *(SFA)* and left profunda femoris *(PF)* arteries. On the left, overlap of the origin of the internal iliac artery obscures this segment. *B,* With 30 degrees of right anterior oblique angulation, the origins of the left external and internal arteries and the bifurcation of the right common femoral artery into the superficial and profunda branches are well seen.

RIGHT VENTRICULOGRAPHY AND PULMONARY ANGIOGRAPHY

Angiography of the right-sided cardiac chambers and the pulmonary vasculature are indicated chiefly for evaluation of congenital heart disease. Thus, they are more commonly performed in the pediatric population than in the adult cardiac catheterization laboratory. However, these procedures are occasionally requested in the adult patient, making it necessary for adult invasive cardiologists to achieve competency in the performance of these procedures and interpretation of the images.

Right Ventriculography. In addition to congenital heart disease, common indications for right ventriculography in the adult patient include diagnosis of right ventricular dysplasia (1) and determination of right ventricular systolic function (2). Right ventriculography is generally not useful to diagnose or quantify tricuspid regurgitation, primarily because the presence of a catheter positioned across the tricuspid valve to perform the right ventriculogram may create artifactual degrees of regurgitation.

A 6 Fr pigtail catheter or a 6 to 7 Fr Berman catheter (a balloon-tipped catheter with multiple side holes and no endhole) are typically used for this purpose. Similar to left ventriculography, the catheter should be positioned within the body of the right ventricle in a stable location without excessive ectopy. A power injector set to inject a volume of 40 mL of contrast at a flow rate of 12 to 14 mL/sec with a rate of increase of 0.8 second and a maximum pressure of 600 pounds per square inch (psi) allows excellent opacification. The radiographic views chosen depend on the indication for the procedure. The right anterior oblique (30-degree) view is useful to diagnose right ventricular dysplasia or to determine right ventricular systolic function. An anteroposterior view is often used for congenital heart disease evaluations and is usually combined with a 90-degree left lateral view when performed in a biplane angiography suite. It is conventional to continue image acquisition well after completing the full contrast injection into the right ventricle to evaluate the pulmonary venous return, the left atrium, and the left ventricle. This technique is known as the "levo" phase of the injection.

Most adult cardiologists are not comfortable interpreting a right ventriculogram, particularly when the diagnosis of arrhythmogenic right ventricular dysplasia is entertained. An example of a normal right ventriculogram, performed in a patient with frequent nonsustained ventricular tachycardia and a structurally normal heart by echocardiography and magnetic resonance imaging, is shown in Video 9-1. This example clearly demonstrates the complex appearance of a normal right ventriculogram with heavy trabeculation and irregular internal contours. The main and branch pulmonary arteries are also clearly seen.

There are no observable features on right ventriculography pathognomonic for arrhythmogenic right ventricular dysplasia. Several findings associated with this disorder, such as apical and/or diaphragmatic dyskinesia with sparing of the right ventricular free wall, are also seen in other conditions that affect the right ventricle including atrial septal defect and biventricular heart failure caused by idiopathic dilated cardiomyopathy (1). Several angiographic aspects reported to be specific for this condition are end-diastolic bulging of the posterior subtricuspid and anterior infundibular walls, and transversally arranged hypertrophic trabeculae separated by deep fissures (1).

Pulmonary Angiography. Similar to right ventriculography, pulmonary angiography is most commonly used in the invasive evaluation of patients with congenital heart disease. This procedure is useful to determine the adequacy of lung perfusion from the pulmonary arteries and diagnoses peripheral pulmonary artery stenosis (Video 9-2), pulmonary arteriovenous malformations (Video 9-3), and patency of surgical conduits and grafts (Video 9-4). The pulmonary valve and outflow tract are clearly imaged by this technique, and in addition to hemodynamic assessment, the technique is useful for the diagnosis of pulmonary valve stenosis (Video 9-5) and pulmonary valve regurgitation, a common consequence of surgical or balloon valvulotomy for congenital pulmonic stenosis or repair of tetralogy of Fallot (Video 9-6). Finally, the levo phase of the pulmonary angiogram can be used to determine the location of the pulmonary veins.

In patients without congenital heart disease, pulmonary angiography may be used to assist the operator perform a trans-septal catheterization because the levo phase of the pulmonary angiogram helps precisely localize the left atrium in the 90-degree left lateral projection (Fig. 9-1). Additional indications for pulmonary angiography include the diagnosis of pulmonary artery dilatation, pulmonic insufficiency, and pulmonary artery vascular malformations. An example of a pulmonary angiogram performed to evaluate pulmonic stenosis in a patient 3 years after a Ross procedure (i.e., transplantation of the patient's pulmonic valve to the aortic position to replace a stenotic aortic valve followed by implantation of a bioprosthetic valve into the pulmonic position) is shown in Video 9-7 and demonstrates narrowing of the entire conduit likely caused by an inflammatory reaction to the bioprosthetic pulmonary valve (3). Although pulmonary angiography may occasionally be performed in the cardiac catheterization laboratory to diagnose pulmonary embolism (Video 9-8), this is more commonly accomplished in the radiology suite by computed tomographic pulmonary angiography or still-frame image acquisition.

To perform this procedure, the operator positions a 6 to 7 F Berman catheter (balloon flotation catheter with multiple side holes and no end hole) in the main pulmonary artery above the pulmonic valve. Power injector settings similar to those used for right ventriculography are appropriate (volume of 40–50 mL of contrast at a flow rate of 12–15 mL/sec with a rate of increase of 0.8 second and a maximum pressure of 800 psi). Image acquisition occurs in the straight anteroposterior projection with the addition of a straight lateral (90 degrees left anterior oblique) if biplane angiography is available. Again, imaging should continue after completing contrast injection to acquire the levo phase (see Video 9-7).

References

1. Daliento L, Rizzoli G, Thiene G, et al: Diagnostic accuracy of right ventriculography in arrhythmogenic right ventricular cardiomyopathy. Am J Cardiol 1990;66:741–745.
2. La Vecchia L, Zanolla L, Varotto L, et al: Reduced right ventricular ejection fraction as a marker for idiopathic dilated cardiomyopathy compared with ischemic left ventricular dysfunction. Am Heart J 2001;142:181–189.
3. Carr-White GS, Kilner PJ, Hon JKF, et al: Incidence, location, pathology, and significance of pulmonary homograft stenosis after the Ross operation. Circulation 2001;104:I-16–I-20.

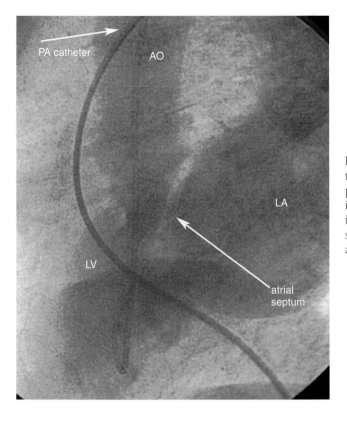

FIGURE 9-1.   A 90-degree left lateral view of the heart during the levo phase of a pulmonary angiogram. This procedure was performed to assist the operator perform a trans-septal catheterization. Note the position of the pulmonary artery *(PA)* catheter in the pulmonary outflow tract. The interatrial septum is clearly seen together with the left atrium *(LA)*, left ventricle *(LV)*, and aorta *(AO)*.

CHAPTER 10

BASIC CORONARY ANGIOGRAPHY

Early efforts at cardiac catheterization focused on patients with congenital and valvular heart disease and consisted primarily of hemodynamic studies, ventriculography and aortography. Coronary angiography was not a part of these early procedures. Injection of contrast directly into a coronary artery was deemed too dangerous and believed likely to cause fatal arrhythmias. Because of this, coronary artery disease remained poorly defined and poorly treated. The field of cardiac catheterization changed dramatically on October 30, 1958, when Dr. F. Mason Sones accidentally performed the first selective coronary angiogram while performing a diagnostic catheterization in a patient with aortic regurgitation. During the procedure, the catheter positioned in the aortic root for aortography inadvertently fell into the right coronary ostium during power injection of 40 mL of ionic contrast (1). Quickly recognizing the error, he aborted the procedure, but about 30 mL of contrast had already been delivered into the right coronary artery. Asystole ensued. Dr. Sones remained levelheaded, instructing the patient to cough repeatedly, thereby generating enough stimulation to resume cardiac action. The patient recovered without event.

A less insightful individual might have viewed the event as a mishap to be avoided, vowing to show greater care in the future. Sones, a true visionary, interpreted the event quite differently; he clearly recognized that his accidental injection proved that selective opacification of human coronary arteries was feasible. Two days later, he successfully performed the first planned selective coronary injection. From that point on, Dr. F. Mason Sones, together with Drs. Melvin Judkins, Kurt Amplatz, and others, refined and developed the technique and catheters for selective coronary angiography that eventually evolved into the safe, routine procedure currently in use.

Current Status of Coronary Angiography. Coronary angiography has become one of the most frequently performed medical procedures, involving about 2 million patients in the United States each year. Selective coronary angiography is the established gold standard for delineation of coronary anatomy and for identifying the presence of luminal obstruction from coronary artery disease. Coronary angiography remains the dominant method for demonstrating coronary luminal obstruction by atheroma or thrombus and for guiding the choice of revascularization procedures. Current techniques easily and safely define vessel dominance and the vascular territories for each artery and, with a resolution of 100 μM, also provide exquisite details of the coronary arteries and its branches. Obstructive coronary disease is often defined by angiography as a greater than 50% diameter narrowing; lesions are generally believed to be "hemodynamically significant" when they narrow the lumen by more than 70%.

Coronary angiography has several limitations. First, and perhaps the most important of these, is the fact that angiography assesses only the arterial lumen. Atherosclerosis is a disease of the arterial wall. A substantial amount of plaque exists before it is evident by angiography. In fact, lumen size is maintained with progressive atherosclerosis by compensatory enlargement of the artery (Glagov phenomenon); lumen encroachment does not occur until atherosclerosis is advanced (Fig. 10-1). Thus, a "normal" coronary angiography does not exclude the presence of coronary artery disease. Even mild degrees of luminal narrowing indicate a fairly sizable atherosclerotic burden. Second, identification of a stenosis depends on the presence of a normal "reference segment" for comparison. In patients with diffuse coronary disease, the arterial lumen diameter may appear uniform on angiography because of the absence of a true "normal" segment, thereby underestimating disease severity. Third, the ability of an angiogram to accurately assess a lesion is dependent on image quality, which, in turn, is dependent on operator technique, patient body habitus, and the degree of vessel tortuosity, lesion eccentricity, or the presence of overlapping segments. Finally, coronary angiography is subject to interpretation; the wide degree of interobserver variability with coronary angiography is well known.

Principles of Coronary Angiography. Given the intrinsic limitations of coronary angiography, it is imperative that the operator strive for the highest quality images. Several important principles underlie the optimal performance of diagnostic coronary angiography. First, it is important to selectively engage the coronary artery, allowing proper filling of the vessel with contrast. Second, the catheter should be positioned coaxial to the artery, and contrast injected at a rate and volume necessary to replace blood with contrast and to allow reflux of contrast into the aorta to ensure imaging of the ostium. Third, each major arterial segment should be imaged in at least two views, 90 degrees apart, and each segment should be free of overlapping vessels. Finally, before slipping off their gloves with a satisfied snap, operators should carefully review the images to be sure that all vessels and arterial segments are seen.

Perfecting injection technique takes a great deal of practice and operator experience. An overly enthusiastic injection of contrast into a relatively small artery may cause myocardial staining and possibly arrhythmia. A weak and inadequate injection causes poor opacification and a "streaming" effect leading to artifacts or missed diagnoses. A prolonged contrast injection increases the risk for bradycardia or ventricular fibrillation, and a noncoaxial catheter position may cause coronary dissection.

Indications and Contraindications for Coronary Angiography. Coronary angiography has numerous indications. In general, coronary angiography is indicated for patients in whom it is necessary to define the coronary anatomy and to diagnose the presence of luminal obstruction. Guidelines for appropriate use of coronary angiography in multiple clinical scenarios including patients with acute myocardial infarction, acute coronary syndromes, stable angina, nonspecific chest pain, valvular and congenital heart disease, heart failure, and other conditions are reviewed in several American College of Cardiology/American Heart Association practice guidelines (2–6).

Coronary angiography is generally contraindicated in patients who do not wish revascularization or who are not candidates for revascularization, or in patients in whom revascularization is not likely to improve quality or duration of life. It is not indicated as a screening test for coronary artery disease in asymptomatic patients or in patients found to have coronary calcium on fluoroscopy or electron beam computed tomography without other indication. Coronary angiography is relatively contraindicated in patients with acute renal failure, active bleeding; unexplained fever; acute stroke; severe, uncontrolled hypertension; severe electrolyte imbalance or metabolic disarray, inability to cooperate; refusal to temporarily rescind a "do not resuscitate" order to allow cardioversion of ventricular fibrillation or other, correctable arrhythmia caused by the procedure; prior anaphylaxis to contrast; prior cholesterol embolization syndrome; severe coagulopathy; and active aortic valve endocarditis. In these situations, the risk-benefit ratio should be carefully considered before proceeding with coronary angiography. Although coronary angiography is a safe procedure, there is the potential for risk; these risks are discussed extensively in Chapter 3.

Contrast Agents. Numerous contrast agents are available for selective coronary angiography (Table 10-1). All contain iodine and densely opacify the artery. The agents differ in terms of osmolality, ionicity, and cost. In general, the low-osmolar, nonionic agents have fewer side effects and are believed to have less renal toxicity than high-osmolar, ionic agents. Gadolinium, a contrast agent used for magnetic resonance imaging, does not contain iodine and has been used with some success for coronary angiography in patients who have had life-threatening anaphylactoid reactions to conventional contrast agents, but it is generally not recommended because it opacifies the arteries poorly and is expensive and is contraindicated in patients with renal failure.

Iodinated contrast agents are associated with several well-known side effects and potential toxicities. Some of these are related to the osmolality and ionicity of the agent, and some are intrinsic to the iodinated compounds. Potential cardiovascular effects include hypotension from vasodilatation, arrhythmia (including ventricular fibrillation or ventricular tachycardia, asystole, and bradycardia), transient ST-segment and T-wave changes on the electrocardiogram, and transient myocardial depression. Anaphylactoid reactions are a rare but well-known potential problem with iodinated contrast. The most common allergic reaction is urticaria, but more serious and life-threatening reactions including bronchospasm, angioedema, laryngospasm, hypotension, and shock may occur. Contrast allergies can be reduced with steroid and antihistamine pretreatment but are not eliminated; therefore, the risk-benefit ratio of coronary angiography in patients who have had a prior severe allergic reaction to contrast should be carefully considered. Central nervous system toxicity including cortical blindness and seizures has been reported.

Renal toxicity, often termed *contrast-induced nephropathy,* is an important clinical concern. Patients with impaired renal function at baseline, diabetes mellitus, and hypovolemia are at increased risk for renal failure from contrast exposure. Many pharmacologic agents and strategies have been proposed to reduce the occurrence of contrast-induced nephropathy, but few have consistently shown benefit (7). Currently, the most effective methods to reduce renal toxicity include limiting the volume of contrast used and hydration with saline. Performance of coronary angiography in a biplane laboratory or, if only a single plane is available, limiting the number of views obtained can greatly reduce the volume of contrast used. In most cases, if carefully done, coronary angiography can be performed with 20 mL or less of contrast, a dose rarely associated with renal failure.

Coronary Catheters. Multiple, preformed catheters are available for performance of selective coronary angiography. In most cases, the standard-sized, Judkins catheters easily engage the artery and result in excellent angiograms. Individual variations in the size and configuration of the aortic root, and location and orientation of the coronary ostia necessitate the use of other sizes or different catheter shapes. Catheters are available in several lumen diameters. The 6 French (Fr) catheters are popular, providing excellent opacification of the coronaries in most cases. Smaller lumen catheters (4 and 5 Fr) are offered but may not allow delivery of an adequate amount of contrast, resulting in poor opacification. Patients with large coronary arteries, high cardiac output, and aortic insufficiency usually need catheters with larger-bore lumens.

Table 10-1.   Contrast Agents for Coronary Angiography

NAME	TYPE OF AGENT	OSMOLALITY	COST
Metrizoate (Isopaque)	Ionic, high osmolar	2100 mOsm	+
Diatrizoate (Hypaque)	Ionic, high osmolar	2016 mOsm	+
Ioxaglate (Hexabrix)	Ionic, low osmolar	600 mOsm	+ + + +
Iohexol (Omnipaque)	Nonionic, low osmolar	862 mOsm	+ +
Iopamidol (Isovue)	Nonionic, low osmolar	796 mOsm	+ +
Iodixanol (Visipaque)	Nonionic, isosmolar	290 mOsm	+ + + +
Gadolinium (Magnevist)	Noniodine containing	1960 mOsm	+ + + +

Important variables to consider when choosing a catheter for selective angiography include the size and shape of the aortic root, orientation of the aortic valve plane, and the location and direction of the coronary ostia (Table 10-2). Cannulation of the coronary ostia in patients with large aortic roots or ascending aortic aneurysms can be particularly challenging requiring large catheters such as the left Judkins 6 (JL-6) or Amplatz left 3 (AL-3). Variations in the aortic valve plane influence catheter selection. The valve plane is often more horizontal in patients with severe chronic obstructive lung disease, whereas patients with marked left ventricular hypertrophy or an unfolded aorta because of advanced age have vertically oriented valve planes (Fig. 10-2 and Video 10-1).

Selective Cannulation of the Left Coronary Artery. From the femoral approach, engagement of the left coronary artery is accomplished in most cases with a JL curve catheter. Usually, this catheter requires no manipulation other than a simple forward push by the operator. The standard-size catheter is a JL-4; the number defines the length of the secondary curve in centimeters. Variations in aortic root size may prevent the JL-4 from selectively engaging the left main stem. For narrow aortic roots, a JL-3.5 can be tried, and for large aortic roots, a JL-5 or a JL-6 is often successful. Many operators use either the anteroposterior (AP) or the left anterior oblique (LAO) projections to selectively cannulate the left coronary artery. If difficulty is encountered, the LAO caudal projection can help determine whether a longer or shorter catheter is required (Fig. 10-3).

Selective angiography of the left coronary vessels may be difficult in the event of a commonly found anomaly where the left main is very short or the ostia of the circumflex and the left anterior descending artery each originate separately from the aorta. Attempts to image both arteries with a single injection usually fail. Instead, it is better to selectively engage and image each artery separately. In this anomaly, the JL-4 catheter usually engages the left anterior descending artery (Fig. 10-4A), and a longer catheter (e.g., a JL-5) successfully engages the left circumflex (see Fig. 10-4B). Alternatively, with the catheter selectively engaged in the left anterior descending artery, rotation of the Judkins catheter in a clockwise fashion may selectively engage the circumflex, whereas a counterclockwise turn moves the catheter from the left circumflex to the left anterior descending artery.

Table 10-2.	**Choice of Catheters for Selective Coronary Angiography**
CATHETER	INDICATION
JR-3.5	RCA if small aortic root
JR-4.0	Default catheter for engaging the RCA
JR-5.0	RCA if large aortic root
AR-1.0	Aberrant origin of RCA, small root
AR-2.0	Aberrant origin of RCA, anomalous vessels or vein grafts
JL-3.0, -3.5	LCA if small aortic root or superior directed left main
JL-4.0	Default catheter for engaging the LCA
JL-5.0	LCA if large aortic root
JL-6.0	LCA if large aortic root
AL-1.0	Aberrant origin of LCA or RCA, small root
AL-2.0	Aberrant origin of LCA or RCA; vein grafts, anomalous vessels
AL-3.0	Aberrant origin of LCA or RCA, large root
MP	Any coronary artery or vein graft
IMA	Internal mammary graft or superiorly directed RCA
RCB	Right coronary bypass grafts, inferiorly directed RCA
LCB	Left coronary bypass grafts

AL, Amplatz left; AR, Amplatz right; IMA, internal mammary artery; JL, Judkins left; JR, Judkins right; LCA, left coronary artery; LCB, left coronary bypass; MP, multipurpose; RCA, right coronary artery; RCB, right coronary bypass.

Common variations in origin or orientation of the left main stem may lead to difficult catheter engagement. Standard JL catheters tend to point superiorly; thus, inferiorly directed left main stems or origins higher than usual from the aortic sinus may prove difficult to engage with this catheter. In such cases, a longer Judkins curve or a left Amplatz (AL) curve may cannulate successfully. In the event of an extreme, superiorly directed left main stem, a shorter catheter (e.g., a JL-3.5) may succeed despite a normal diameter aortic root. Similarly, the "C" curve, available as an angioplasty guide catheter, may prove highly successful. Posteriorly directed left main stems are commonly encountered; these usually require an AL catheter.

Standard JL catheters are not as useful from the brachial or radial approach. From a left brachial approach, the left coronary artery tends to require a more superiorly directed catheter such as a JL-3.5 or a "C" curve guide catheter. From the right radial or right brachial approach, the "C" curves often prove successful; many operators also use AL curves or one of the specialty catheters specifically designed for radial approach.

Selective Engagement of the Right Coronary Artery. The right coronary artery is engaged in a straight LAO view by turning a right Judkins catheter (JR-4) in a clockwise rotation. This artery requires more operator skill to engage than the left coronary artery. In the event of a large, dilated aorta, a JR-5 catheter is used; similarly, a JR-3.5 can be used for small aortas. When the right coronary artery is not found in the usual location, it is likely aberrant in origin typically located from a high and anterior position on the aorta. These may prove challenging to engage and usually require either less clockwise turn or an AR or AL curve. The AR catheter (usually an AR-2) is engaged similar to a JR catheter using a gentle clockwise rotation. AL catheters (usually AL-1 or AL-2) require a greater degree of care and skill to engage. To engage a right coronary artery with an AL catheter, the operator first brings the catheter tip to the level of the coronary ostium and gently turns the catheter clockwise. Great care must be used because this catheter has a tendency to lurch uncontrollably into the coronary artery potentially dissecting the vessel. In addition, once engaged, pulling back on the catheter tends to cause the tip to dive forward. For this reason, when removing the AL catheter from the right coronary artery, the operator should push down and/or turn the catheter to disengage it first before withdrawing it from the aorta.

Most right coronary arteries originate horizontally from the aorta or with a slight superior direction. Both the inferiorly and superiorly directed right coronary ostium may be quite challenging to engage with a standard Judkins catheter. The superiorly directed ostium can sometimes be engaged with an internal mammary artery catheter, whereas the inferiorly directed ostium can be cannulated with either a right coronary bypass catheter or an Amplatz catheter.

Catheter Tip Pressure Waveforms. Immediately on engaging a coronary artery and before performance of angiography, the operator should carefully examine the pressure waveform generated from the catheter tip. Normally, the pressure waveform appears as a typical aortic pressure waveform. Two abnormalities in the pressure waveform are important to recognize: damping and ventricularization. Pressure "damping" refers to a decline in the systolic pressure and a loss of the usual features of an arterial pressure waveform. The term *ventricularization* describes a decline in the diastolic pressure and a shift in appearance from the usual arterial waveform to a ventricular waveform. More typically, the pressure trace has features of both (Fig. 10-5). Damping and ventricularization have similar causes (Table 10-3); they imply plugging of the coronary lumen with the catheter tip most commonly because of obstructive disease of the coronary ostium or selective engagement of an artery smaller than the catheter such as the conus branch of the right coronary artery. Before proceeding with contrast injection, the angiographer should first determine the cause. Injection of contrast into a catheter with a damped or ventricularized pressure tracing might lead to a serious complication such as arrhythmia or dissection of the proximal artery (Videos 10-2 and 10-3). Thus, the angiographer should be constantly vigilant for this finding. When observed, the catheter

Table 10-3.	Causes of Damping or Ventricularization, or Both, of Catheter Pressure Waveform

During Engagement of the Right Coronary Artery (RCA)

1. Atherosclerotic disease of the ostium of the RCA

2. Catheter-induced spasm of the coronary artery

3. Selective engagement of the conus branch of the RCA

4. Total occlusion of the RCA

5. Engagement of a small, nondominant artery

During Engagement of the Left Coronary Artery

1. Atherosclerotic disease of the ostium of the left main stem

2. Deep seating of the catheter and selective engagement of either the left anterior descending artery or left circumflex artery

During Engagement of Either Coronary Artery

1. Presence of a small-caliber artery with match in size between the diameter of the catheter and the coronary artery

2. Kinking of the catheter during catheter manipulation

3. Malposition of the catheter against the wall of the aorta

4. Presence of thrombus or air bubble in the catheter

may be withdrawn into the aortic root and contrast injected into the aortic cusp to determine whether there is ostial disease. Alternatively, a small amount of contrast may be carefully injected into the damped coronary catheter to determine the cause.

Normal Coronary Anatomy. In the majority of individuals, the major epicardial coronary arteries follow fairly predictable patterns. The vascular distributions of the specific branches, however, vary greatly between individuals.

Normally, a single right coronary artery emanates from the right sinus of Valsalva and courses along the atrioventricular groove, providing first a conus branch to the right ventricular outflow tract, then right ventricular marginal arteries to the right ventricular myocardium. In a right-dominant circulation (roughly 60–70% of patients), the right coronary artery bifurcates at the bottom of the atrioventricular groove into the posterior descending artery and the posterolateral artery. The posterior descending artery runs along the interventricular groove supplying septal perforators to the inferior septum.

The left main coronary artery originates from the anterior (or left) sinus of Valsalva and quickly branches into the posteriorly directed left circumflex artery and the anteriorly directed left anterior descending artery. In about 20% of patients, a clearly defined third branch emanates from the left main stem between these two arteries and is called the *ramus intermedius*. The left anterior descending artery runs along the anterior aspect of the atrioventricular groove, supplying septal perforators to the septum and diagonal branches to the lateral wall of the heart, ultimately terminating in apical branches supplying the apex of the left ventricle. The circumflex artery runs posteriorly in the atrioventricular groove supplying left atrial branches to the left atrium and obtuse marginal arteries to the lateral wall of the left ventricle. In the event of a left-dominant circulation (roughly 20% of patients), the circumflex continues and supplies a left posterior descending artery and left posterolateral branches. Variations in the specific branches are common between individuals. In addition, many different coronary anomalies have been described and are discussed in Chapter 14. Examples of the normal coronary distribution for right-dominant and left-dominant circulations are shown in Figures 10-6 and 10-7.

Angiographic Views. The complex and serpiginous array of vessels constituting the coronary arterial circulation mandates the need for multiple angiographic views to visualize all segments free of overlap and foreshortening. The nomenclature used to define these views is based on the position of the image intensifier relative to the midline of the supine patient (Fig. 10-8). The X-ray source lies under the patient, and the image intensifier typically lies above the patient. When the image intensifier is directly above the patient's chest, the camera is in the AP position. The angle relative to the midline defines the view. For example, if the image intensifier is 30 degrees to the left of midline, this is known as 30 degrees LAO. Positioning the image intensifier toward the head is known as *cranial angulation,* and positioning the image intensifier toward the feet is known as *caudal angulation.*

The right coronary artery is usually imaged in two views: the LAO and the right anterior oblique (RAO) projection. Typical angles are about 45 degrees LAO with 10 to 15 degrees of cranial angulation and 35 to 45 degrees straight RAO. The RAO projection clearly images the midportion of the right coronary artery demonstrating the origins of the right ventricular marginal branches; this view also lays out the extent of the posterior descending artery. The RAO view does not provide a clear view of the ostium of the right coronary artery or of the distal bifurcation of the posterolateral and posterior descending artery. The LAO projection provides a better view of the right coronary ostium; in addition, this view shows the midsegments well and demonstrates the distal bifurcation of the posterolateral and posterior descending artery or "crux." Adding cranial angulation can eliminate overlap of these two branches and improve the visualization of the distal bifurcation. In difficult cases with significant overlap, an AP cranial view may more clearly define this area. Alternative views include the RAO cranial or RAO caudal view. Finally, the lateral (or 90-degree LAO) view of the right coronary artery is an excellent adjunctive view for imaging the midportion of the right coronary artery and for discriminating the posterior descending artery from the posterolateral branch (Fig. 10-9).

There are usually five standard views of the left coronary artery. The RAO caudal view (20–30 degrees RAO and 20–30 degrees caudal) is an excellent view of the circumflex and obtuse marginal branches, the distal left main, and the ostium and proximal segment of the left anterior descending artery. This view significantly foreshortens the mid and distal segments of the left anterior descending artery obscuring the origins of the diagonals. The RAO cranial views (5–10 degrees RAO and 30–40 degrees cranial or 30 degrees RAO and 30 degrees cranial) are best for the mid and distal segments of the left anterior descending artery and clearly display the origins of the diagonal arteries. In general, the RAO cranial projection is not useful for the circumflex because of foreshortening artifact; however, in left-dominant circulations, the RAO cranial view provides a good view of the very distal, lower obtuse marginal branches and of the left posterior descending artery. The LAO caudal view (50 degrees LAO and 20–30 degrees caudal) is an important view for the distal left main stem and the proximal segments of the left anterior descending artery, the ramus intermedius, and the circumflex. It provides clear definition of the body of the circumflex and the origin of the marginal branches. The LAO cranial view (50–60 degrees LAO and 20–30 degrees cranial) demonstrates the mid and distal segments of the left anterior descending artery and the origin of the diagonals. Importantly, it is also one of the few views clearly depicting the ostium of the left main artery. The proximal portion of the left anterior descending artery is usually foreshortened in this view, and the operator must be careful that there is not overlap of the circumflex and proximal left anterior descending artery; additional LAO angulation corrects this problem. The lateral view (90-degree LAO) is best for the mid and distal segments of the left anterior descending artery and for the circumflex.

Additional views help image some problematic segments of the left coronary artery. The AP caudal view (straight AP with 20–30 degrees caudal) may be useful for the proximal left anterior descending artery, the ostium of the left main stem, and for the circumflex and marginal arteries. The AP cranial view (straight AP with 20–40 degrees cranial) may show segments of the proximal left anterior descending artery not well seen in the more standard RAO cranial views and may also more clearly depict the origin of the diagonal branches. Over-rotation of the lateral view (i.e., 100 or 110 degrees of LAO) may be helpful to remove diagonals from overlapping segments of the left anterior descending artery.

References

1. Ryan TJ: The coronary angiogram and its seminal contributions to cardiovascular medicine over five decades. Circulation 2002;106:752–756.
2. Scanlon PJ, Faxon DP, Audet AM, et al: ACC/AHA guidelines for coronary angiography: A report of the American College of Cardiology/American Heart Association Task Force on Practice Guidelines (Committee on Coronary Angiography). J Am Coll Cardiol 1999;33:1756–1824.
3. Antman EM, Anbe DT, Armstrong PW, et al: ACC/AHA guidelines for the management of patients with ST-elevation myocardial infarction: A report of the American College of Cardiology/American Heart Association Task Force on Practice Guidelines (Committee to Revise the 1999 Guidelines for the Management of Patients With Acute Myocardial Infarction). Circulation 2004; 110:e82–e293.
4. Bonow RO, Carabello BA, Chatterjee K, et al: ACC/AHA 2006 guidelines for the management of patients with valvular heart disease: A report of the American College of Cardiology/American Heart Association Task Force on Practice Guidelines (Writing Committee to Develop Guidelines for the Management of Patients With Valvular Heart Disease). J Am Coll Cardiol 2006;48:e1–e148.
5. Anderson JL, Adams CD, Antman EM, et al: ACC/AHA 2007 guidelines for the management of patients with unstable angina/non–ST-elevation myocardial infarction: A report of the American College of Cardiology/American Heart Association Task Force on Practice Guidelines (Writing Committee to Revise the 2002 Guidelines for the Management of Patients With Unstable Angina/Non–ST-Elevation Myocardial Infarction): Developed in collaboration with the American College of Emergency Physicians, American College of Physicians, Society for Academic Emergency Medicine, Society for Cardiovascular Angiography and Interventions, and Society of Thoracic Surgeons. J Am Coll Cardiol 2007;50:e1–e157.
6. Gibbons RJ, Abrams J, Chatterjee K, et al: ACC/AHA 2002 guideline update for the management of patients with chronic stable angina: A report of the American College of Cardiology/American Heart Association Task Force on Practice Guidelines (Committee to Update the 1999 Guidelines for the Management of Patients with Chronic Stable Angina). 2002. Circulation 2003;107:149–158.
7. Schweiger MJ, Chambers CE, Davidson CJ, et al: Prevention of contrast induced nephropathy: Recommendations for the high risk patient undergoing cardiovascular procedures. Catheter Cardiovasc Interv 2007;69:135–140.

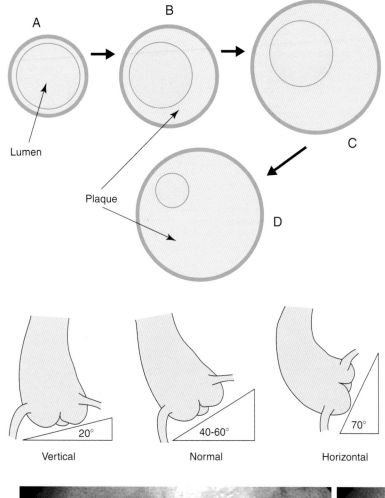

FIGURE 10-1. Atherosclerosis is a disease of the vessel wall. With progressive plaque accumulation, (A,B) the entire vessel grows and initially, the lumen size is maintained. This process is known as the *Glagov phenomenon,* or positive vessel remodeling, and explains why an artery may appear normal by angiography despite the presence of significant atherosclerosis in the arterial wall (C). Lumen encroachment does not occur until the disease is advanced (D).

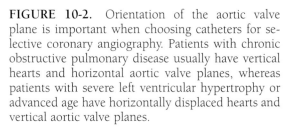

FIGURE 10-2. Orientation of the aortic valve plane is important when choosing catheters for selective coronary angiography. Patients with chronic obstructive pulmonary disease usually have vertical hearts and horizontal aortic valve planes, whereas patients with severe left ventricular hypertrophy or advanced age have horizontally displaced hearts and vertical aortic valve planes.

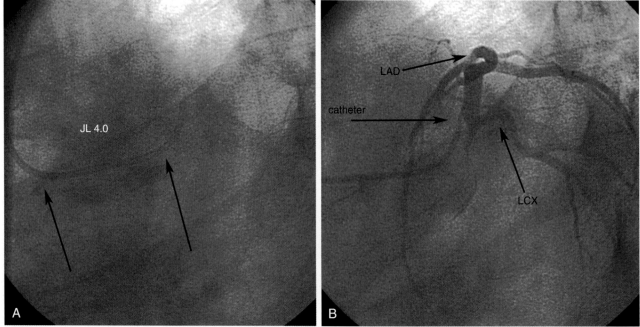

FIGURE 10-3. The left anterior oblique view with caudal angulation is helpful when choosing a Judkins left (JL) catheter. *A,* The number defining the catheter represents the length, in centimeters, of the catheter segment shown by the *arrows.* The goal should be coaxial alignment in the left main stem. A Judkins catheter too short for the left main stem will point toward the left anterior descending artery *(LAD)* (B), whereas an excessively long catheter will point toward the circumflex artery *(LCX).*

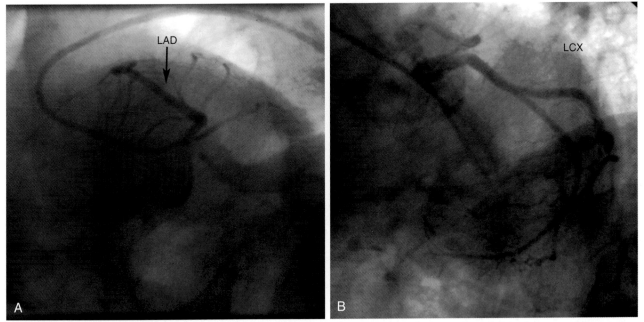

FIGURE 10-4. Left anterior oblique view with caudal angulation in a patient with a very short left main stem. A JL-4 catheter selectively engages the left anterior descending artery *(LAD)* *(A)*, whereas the longer JL-5 catheter selectively engages the left circumflex *(LCX)* *(B)*. JL, left Judkins.

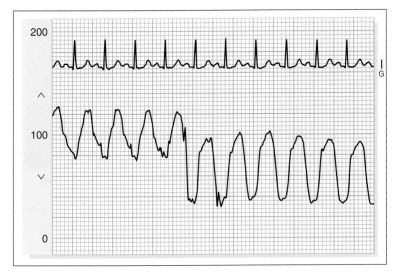

FIGURE 10-5. Example of damping and ventricularization of the catheter pressure waveform.

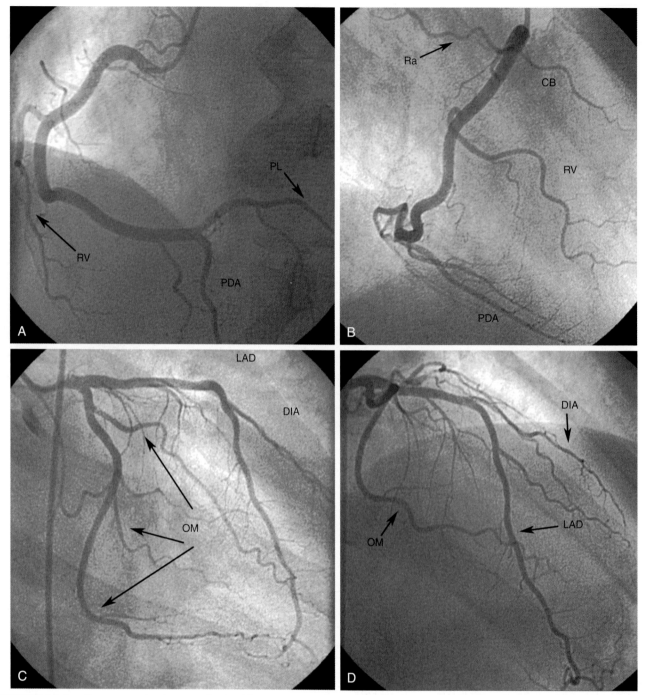

FIGURE 10-6.   Representative images obtained in a patient with angiographic normal, right-dominant circulation. *A,* The right coronary artery is shown in a left anterior oblique projection and *(B)* a right anterior oblique projection. *C,* The left coronary artery is shown in a right anterior oblique with caudal angulation, *(D)* a right anterior oblique with cranial angulation,

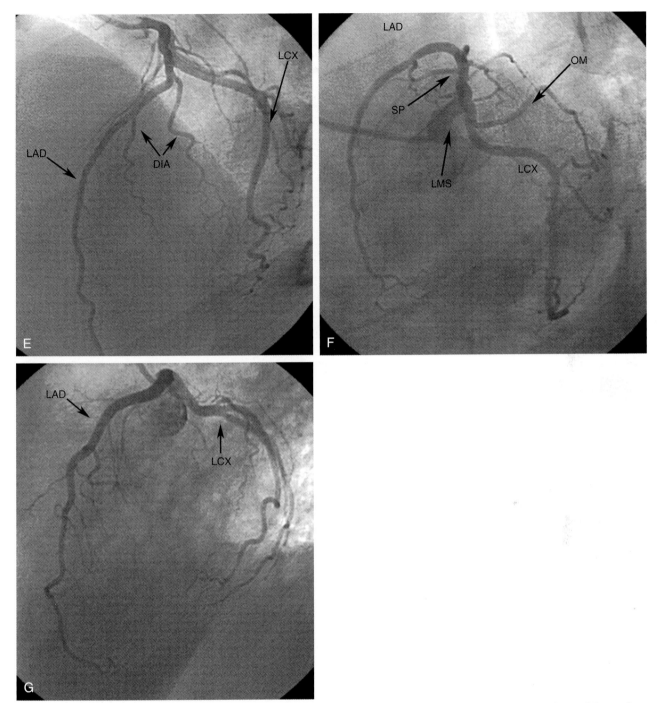

FIGURE 10-6. cont'd (E) a left anterior oblique with cranial angulation, (F) a left anterior oblique with caudal angulation, and (G) a 90-degree left lateral projection. CB, conus branch; DIA, diagonal arteries; LAD, left anterior descending artery; LCX, left circumflex artery; LMS, left main stem; OM, obtuse marginal branches; PDA, posterior descending artery; PL, posterolateral branch; Ra, right atrial branch; RV, right ventricular marginal branch; SP, septal perforators.

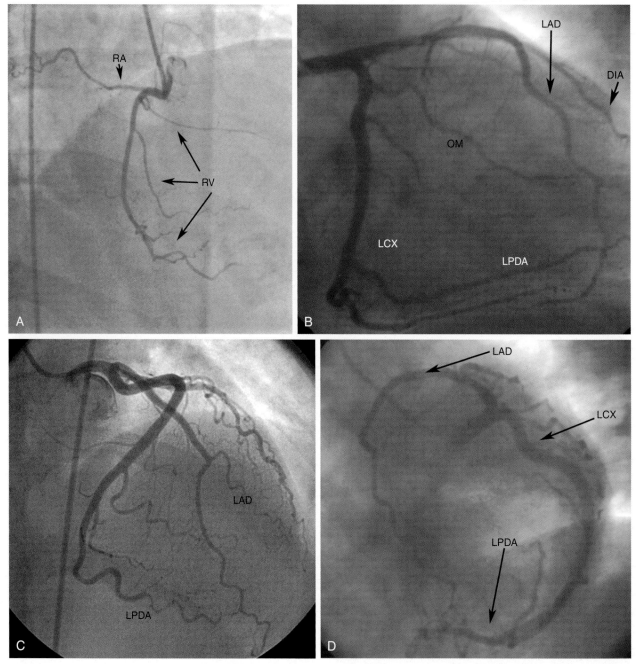

FIGURE 10-7.   Representative images obtained in a patient with angiographic normal, left-dominant circulation. *A,* The right coronary artery is shown in a right anterior oblique projection. *B,* The left coronary artery is shown in a right anterior oblique with caudal angulation, (*C*) a right anterior oblique with cranial angulation, and (*D*) a left anterior oblique with caudal angulation. DIA, diagonal arteries; LAD, left anterior descending artery; LCX, left circumflex artery; LPDA, left posterior descending artery; OM, obtuse marginal branches; RA, right atrial branch; RV, right ventricular marginal branch; SP, septal perforators.

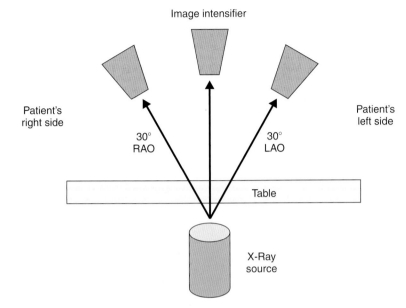

Image intensifier

Patient's right side

Patient's left side

30° RAO

30° LAO

Table

X-Ray source

FIGURE 10-8. Schematic diagram demonstrating the position of the radiation source and image intensifier relative to the patient. Radiographic projections are described in terms of the relative position of the image intensifier to the patient. For example, with the patient lying on his or her back, rotation of the image intensifier toward the patient's right is described as the right anterior oblique (RAO) view, whereas rotation to the patient's left is known as the left anterior oblique (LAO) view. Tilting the image intensifier toward the head is described as cranial angulation, and tilting the image intensifier toward the feet is caudal angulation.

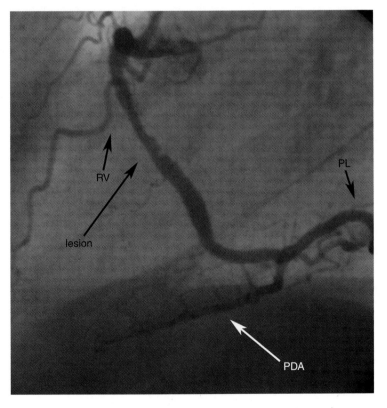

RV

lesion

PL

PDA

FIGURE 10-9. This is a 90-degree left lateral projection of the right coronary artery. Note the moderate stenosis in the midportion of the right coronary artery. This projection is especially helpful to image this segment free of overlap from right ventricular marginal arteries. PDA, posterior descending artery; PL, posterolateral branch; RV, right ventricular marginal artery.

CHAPTER 11

ISCHEMIC HEART DISEASE:
CORONARY PHYSIOLOGY AND MANIFESTATIONS OF CORONARY ATHEROSCLEROSIS

In the United States, most cardiac catheterization procedures consist of coronary angiography performed to evaluate known or suspected ischemic heart disease. Reconciling the findings on coronary angiography with a given patient's syndrome requires a thorough understanding of coronary physiology and the various manifestations of coronary atherosclerosis.

Coronary Physiology. Coronary blood flow is determined primarily by myocardial oxygen consumption, which, in turn, increases with increases in wall tension, heart rate, and contractility. During physical exertion, myocardial oxygen consumption may increase four to five times over basal levels. Because the highly efficient myocardium extracts nearly all of the oxygen delivered to it, any increase in myocardial oxygen demand requires an increase in blood flow.

Coronary blood flow is regulated by a complex system and is dependent primarily on the driving pressure and the resistance of the coronary vessels. Extravascular coronary compression from left ventricular contractile force impairs flow during systole in the left coronary artery such that maximum flow occurs during early diastole. Right ventricular forces are much less than left ventricular contraction; thus, coronary flow is fairly even during both diastole and systole in the right coronary artery.

Myocardial blood flow at rest is fairly constant despite fluctuations in blood pressure. This concept is known as *autoregulation,* a term used to describe the ability of the heart to maintain relatively constant blood flow over a wide range of coronary perfusion pressures. Normally, perfusion is maintained when the mean aortic pressure is 45 to 150 mm Hg. Outside of this range, coronary blood flow is directly dependent on pressure.

The major variable controlling coronary blood flow is coronary vascular resistance. The epicardial coronary arteries are primarily conductance vessels and account for only 5% of total coronary vascular resistance. It is the small, intramyocardial arterioles less than 300 μm that account for 95% of the resistance across the coronary bed and vessels less than 100 μm account for 50% of the total coronary resistance. These resistance vessels are the major determinant of coronary blood flow, and they, in turn, are influenced by the endothelium (via nitric oxide, prostaglandins, and endothelin), metabolites (adenosine, hypoxia, and hypercapnia), and neurohormonal mechanisms.

When coronary atherosclerosis develops and begins to impinge on the lumen, the resistance of the conductance vessel increases and pressure declines across the stenosis. Because of autoregulation, blood flow will be maintained by reducing resistance in the small arterioles in the heart. Eventually, with progressive luminal encroachment and further decline in pressure across the stenosis, recruitment of resistance vessels is maximized and no further increase in coronary blood flow can occur. Although this may maintain adequate blood flow at rest, any increase in myocardial oxygen demand will be unable to be met by an increase in blood flow resulting in ischemia. With the development of a severe stenosis, autoregulation is exhausted and blood flow becomes dependent on driving pressure; resting flow may be compromised causing ischemia even in the resting state. Coronary flow reserve describes the amount of additional blood flow that can be supplied to the heart. The absence of coronary flow reserve implies maximal vasodilation of the resistance vessels.

In carefully performed experimental models, abnormalities of flow reserve become evident when stenosis severity narrows the lumen more than 70%. Human atherosclerotic lesions are quite different from these idealized models and are often eccentric and highly complex. Therefore, clinicians cannot rely solely on an angiographic estimate of stenosis severity to decide whether an atherosclerotic lesion is severe enough to cause limitation in flow and ischemia. This is particularly relevant for lesions of moderate (40–70%) severity, long lesions, or tandem lesions. In such cases, coronary flow reserve can be directly measured in the cardiac catheterization laboratory to assist the clinician in determining the hemodynamic significance of a lesion.

Several invasive techniques for assessment of coronary flow reserve have been developed. Initial efforts used the Doppler method, using a 0.014-inch wire outfitted with an ultrasound crystal at its tip. Average peak blood flow velocity is measured at rest (normal 15–30 cm/sec) and again during maximal hyperemia induced pharmacologically with adenosine (1, 2). This technique provides an estimate of absolute flow reserve, defined as the ratio of hyperemic flow in a stenotic artery to resting flow in the same artery; the normal value is greater than 2.0. Abnormal coronary flow reserve indicates full recruitment of the resistance vessels consistent with a hemodynamically significant stenosis. However, absolute flow reserve may also be abnormal if abnormalities of the microcirculation occur. This may occur in the setting of prior myocardial infarction, left ventricular hypertrophy, and diabetes mellitus. Furthermore, this technique is dependent on loading conditions and heart rate, and the Doppler method requires a reliable, high-quality Doppler signal that may not be obtainable in patients with tortuous coronary arteries or who have lesions near branch points. Because of these limitations, this technique is not routinely used in the cardiac catheterization laboratory for this purpose and has been supplanted by the measurement of fractional flow reserve (FFR).

FFR is another method of assessing the significance of intermediate coronary stenosis. Unlike Doppler methodology, it is independent of loading conditions and microvascular disease. This technique has been well validated in humans and is an easy method of determining the significance of a stenosis (3–6).

FFR is a pressure-based method for determining coronary flow reserve and is derived from the relation among pressure, flow, and resistance. The term *fractional flow reserve* (FFR) describes the ratio between the maximum myocardial blood flow in the presence of a stenosis to the theoretical maximum flow in the absence of a stenosis (i.e., the normal artery). It is easily calculated as follows:

FFR = mean hyperemic distal intracoronary pressure ÷ mean hyperemic arterial pressure

A normal FFR is 1.0. Coronary stenosis found to have a FFR less than 0.75 is associated with ischemia and is thus classified as "hemodynamically significant."

FFR is easily performed in the cardiac catheterization laboratory using a proprietary angioplasty guide wire fitted with a pressure transducer several centimeters from the wire tip. After inserting a guide catheter and administering heparin (50 U/kg), the pressure wire is attached to a computerized console, and the system is zeroed and calibrated. After ensuring that the wire transducer and catheter tip pressures are identical, the pressure wire transducer is advanced beyond the stenosis and maximal hyperemia is induced. As described in the earlier formula, FFR is simply calculated as the ratio of the distal pressure to aortic pressure during maximal hyperemia.

Maximal hyperemia can be induced by one of several methods. The easiest is to inject adenosine (30–60 mcg for the right coronary artery and 60–100 mcg for the left coronary artery) directly into the coronary artery via the guide catheter. Peak hyperemia is present after about 5 seconds and quickly dissipates. Alternatively, a more sustained hyperemia can be provoked by using intravenous infusion of adenosine (140 mcg/kg/min) via a large vein; however, this adds significant cost to the procedure. With either technique, maximal hyperemia is defined as the nadir of the mean pressures.

FFR is routinely used as an adjunct to angiography primarily to determine the hemodynamic significance of moderate (40–70%) coronary lesions. It is also helpful to determine the significance of lesions that are difficult to image by angiography. Examples include eccentric plaques and lesions within tortuous segments, in areas with foreshortening artifact, or overlapped by branch vessels. Figures 11-1 and 11-2 show examples of the use of FFR in clinical practice.

Manifestations of Coronary Atherosclerosis. Coronary angiography is traditionally considered the gold standard for diagnosing coronary artery disease. The myriad of angiographic manifestations of coronary atherosclerosis exceeds the scope of this discussion; however, several frequently observed findings have been reported.

Notably, coronary atherosclerosis is already well established by the time it is apparent on angiography. In the early stages of coronary atherosclerosis, the lumen is maintained despite progressive atherosclerosis by compensatory enlargement of the artery (7, 8). Because angiography assesses only the arterial lumen, this phase of atherosclerosis escapes detection by angiography. As described in Chapter 10, because of the Glagov phenomenon, the lumen is maintained despite the presence of atherosclerosis in the arterial wall (Fig. 11-3). Luminal encroachment becomes apparent only when atherosclerosis is advanced. For this reason, a "normal" coronary angiogram does not exclude the presence of coronary artery disease. Even mild degrees of luminal narrowing imply a fairly sizable atherosclerotic burden. Thus, early detection of coronary atherosclerosis requires imaging of the arterial wall using techniques such as intravascular ultrasound (Fig. 11-4).

With the understanding that coronary atherosclerosis is generally a diffuse process and that angiographically "normal" segments may have atherosclerosis, coronary lesions are often described as being either "focal" if they narrow a defined segment or diffuse if the luminal encroachment involves multiple contiguous segments (Figs. 11-5 and 11-6). This designation is arbitrary and highly subject to interpretation but serves some descriptive value when determining suitability for revascularization procedures. For instance, diffuse atherosclerosis may affect long sections of the artery and is more difficult to revascularize. Obliterative disease represents an extreme version of diffuse involvement (Fig. 11-7).

Coronary lesions can be located anywhere along the course of the artery. Disease of the ostium of the coronary artery may also reflect atheroma of the aortic wall (Fig. 11-8). These lesions are sometimes difficult to diagnose on angiography because they may be masked by reflux of contrast or an overlapping catheter. Coronary lesions also have a tendency to affect bifurcations of major branches. These also can be challenging to image properly and are technically difficult to manage with percutaneous approaches (Fig. 11-9).

The nature of the atherosclerotic plaque is best appreciated by intravascular ultrasound. However, some characteristics are interpretable on angiography. Concentric plaques are easier to treat percutaneously, whereas eccentric plaques have a greater rate of dissection with balloon angioplasty. Stable plaques typically have a smooth appearance, whereas the plaques associated with acute coronary syndromes (unstable angina or acute myocardial infarction) are eccentric, bulky lesions with irregular borders (Fig. 11-10). One of the hallmarks of the acute coronary syndrome is ulceration of an atherosclerotic plaque. This finding may be observed on angiography as a crater of contrast within an area of plaque (Fig. 11-11).

Determining the severity of coronary artery disease is somewhat arbitrary and highly subjective. Quantitative angiographic analysis provides precise measurements of the lumen and stenosis severity but is a tedious process used primarily for research purposes. Stenosis severity often reported by clinicians performing coronary angiography is based solely on visual assessment by comparing a "normal segment" with a diseased segment. It is probably more accurate to describe the results of angiography as showing either no, mild, moderate, or severe luminal obstruction rather than assign a percentage stenosis implying that an actual measurement was made. Typically, these visual estimations overstate stenosis severity. The wide interobserver variability of coronary angiography is well known.

Coronary Collaterals. Coronary collaterals are congenitally established channels that connect epicardial coronary arteries. Collateral channels exist normally, and increase in both size and number in the presence of chronic ischemic heart disease. During acute coronary occlusion, existing collaterals are vital for limiting infarct size, maintaining myocardial viability, and preserving left ventricular function. In the first 12 hours of acute infarction, coronary collaterals are rarely visible by angiography. Only about 5% of patients demonstrate well-developed collaterals, and less than 50% have any angiographic evidence of collateral vessels during this time frame. The extent of collateral development in patients with chronic coronary disease relates to the severity of the underlying stenosis. With persistent occlusion, angiographic collaterals become more apparent such that nearly all patients with chronic coronary occlusion demonstrate angiographic collaterals, and 90% of patients with chronic stable angina and severely narrowed arteries exhibit "recruitable" collaterals.

Although collateral vessels can be easily seen by angiography, these conduits vary in size and many channels are less than the 100-μm limit of resolution of angiography. Therefore, inability to image collaterals by angiography does not necessarily imply their absence. Collaterals often fill the epicardial vessel more slowly. For this reason, it is important to continue image acquisition well after the supplying artery is injected to adequately assess collateral vessels. Administration of nitrates may enhance the angiographic appearance of collateral vessels. This technique may be helpful when a planned revascularization procedure requires clear definition of the status of the target vessel.

Grading systems have been devised in an effort to quantify the extent of collaterals. Angiographic collaterals are classified as *grade 0* if there is an occluded artery and no angiographic visible collateral channels observed, *grade I* if there is only filling of branches of the occluded artery, *grade II* if there is partial filling of the occluded artery, and *grade III* if complete filling of the occluded artery is observed (9). Notably, angiographic collaterals represent epicardial conduits, and their presence does not necessarily imply adequate myocardial tissue perfusion. This information can be determined only by techniques such as nuclear perfusion imaging or myocardial contrast echocardiography.

Collaterals follow predictable patterns. Usually, the epicardial arteries adjacent to or providing overlapping circulation with the occluded artery become the "supply" artery. For example, the posterior descending artery and left anterior descending artery both supply septal perforators. In the event of total occlusion of one of these two vessels, collaterals may arise from the patent artery via the septal perforators to reconstitute the other, occluded artery. Note that collaterals may arise from multiple sources; it is not always possible to determine which artery supplies the majority of the collaterals. The term *bridging* collaterals is often used to describe collaterals emanating from the site of the occlusion and reconstituting the distal portion of the same artery. They have a characteristic "spider-web" appearance and represent dilated vasovasorum (Fig. 11-12).

Commonly observed collateral patterns for occluded dominant right coronary, left circumflex artery, and left anterior descending artery are listed in Table 11-1, with schematic diagrams of these patterns shown in Figures 11-13 through 11-15. Examples of some of these common collateral patterns are shown in Videos 11-1 through 11-8.

Table 11-1.	Angiographic Patterns of Collaterals

Occluded RCA

Right to Right

RV marginal to RV marginal

Conus artery to AV nodal artery (Kugel's artery)

Conus artery to posterolateral branch

Left to Right

LAD to PDA via septum or via the apex

LCX or OM to the posterolateral branch

LAD to RV marginal

Occluded LCX

Left to Left

OM to OM

Diagonal to OM

Right to Left

Conus to LCX

Posterolateral to OM

PDA to Distal LCX

Atrial branch to atrial branch

Occluded LAD

Left to Left

Septal to septal

Diagonal to LAD

OM to LAD

Right to Left

RV marginal to LAD

PDA to LAD via apex or via septum

Conus to LAD

AV, atrioventricular; LAD, left anterior descending; LCX, left circumflex; OM, obtuse marginal; PDA, posterior descending artery; RCA, right coronary artery; RV, right ventricular.

References

1. Miller DD, Donohue TJ, Younis LT: Correlation of pharmacological Tc-sestamibi myocardial perfusion imaging with poststenotic coronary flow reserve in patients with angiographically intermediate coronary artery stenoses. Circulation 1994;89:2150–2160.
2. Joye JD, Schulman DS, Lasorda D, et al: Intracoronary Doppler guide wire versus stress single-photon emission computed tomographic thallium-201 imaging in assessment of intermediate coronary stenoses. J Am Coll Cardiol 1994;24:940–947.
3. Pijls NHJ, Van Gelder B, Van der Voort P, et al: Fractional flow reserve: A useful index to evaluate the influence of an epicardial coronary stenosis on myocardial blood flow. Circulation 1995;92:3183–3193.
4. De Bruyne B, Baudhuin T, Melin JA, et al: Coronary flow reserve calculated from pressure measurements in humans. Validation with PET. Circulation 1994;89:1013–1022.
5. Pijls NHJ, de Bruyne B, Peels K, et al: Measurement of fractional flow reserve to assess the functional severity of coronary artery stenoses. N Engl J Med 1996;334:1703–1708.
6. Pijls NH, van Son JA, Kirkeeide RL, et al: Experimental basis of determining maximum coronary, myocardial, and collateral blood flow by pressure measurements for assessing functional stenosis severity before and after percutaneous transluminal coronary angioplasty. Circulation 1993;87:1354–1367.

7. Glagov S, Weisenberg E, Zarins CK, et al: Compensatory enlargement of human atherosclerotic coronary arteries. N Engl J Med 1987;316:1371–1375.
8. Nissen SE, Yock P: Intravascular ultrasound. Novel pathophysiologic insights and current clinical applications. Circulation 2001;103:604–616.
9. Cohen M, Rentrop KP: Limitation of myocardial ischemia by collateral circulation during sudden controlled coronary artery occlusion in human subjects: A prospective study. Circulation 1986;74:469–476.

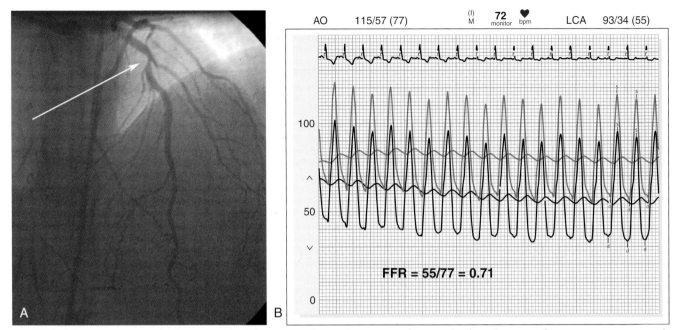

FIGURE 11-1. Example of a lesion in the left anterior descending artery (*A, arrow*) of unclear significance in a patient with an anginal syndrome. *B,* Fractional flow reserve (*FFR*) was performed using intracoronary adenosine and was determined to be 0.71, which is consistent with a significant stenosis.

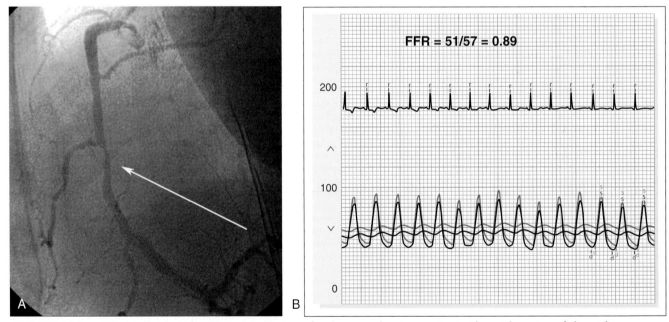

FIGURE 11-2. This angiogram demonstrates a lesion of at least moderate severity in the midportion of the right coronary artery (*A, arrow*) in a patient with a chest pain syndrome. *B,* Fractional flow reserve (*FFR*) was performed using intracoronary adenosine and was determined to be 0.89, and thus was not a significant stenosis.

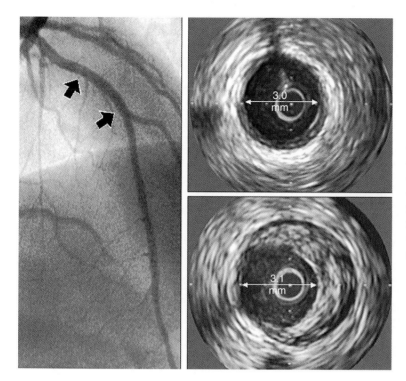

FIGURE 11-3. Demonstration of the Glagov phenomenon. Angiography shows a fairly uniform lumen in the left anterior descending artery. Intravascular ultrasound performed at two different sites (*arrows*) reveals that, although the lumen is the same size, significant plaque is present in the arterial wall at the more distal site.
(Reproduced from Nissen and Yock (8) by permission.)

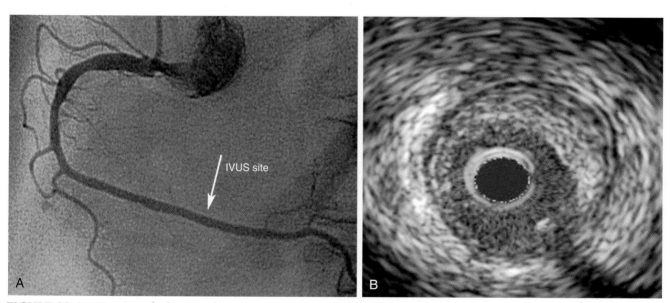

FIGURE 11-4.   Despite a fairly normal appearance on angiography (*A*), a substantial atherosclerotic plaque is present within the arterial wall as shown by intravascular ultrasound (IVUS) (*B*). IVUS, intravascular ultrasound.

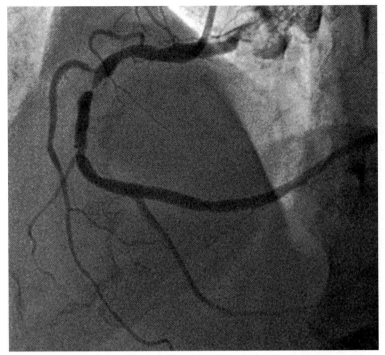

FIGURE 11-5.   An example of a focal, smooth stenosis in the right coronary artery causing stable, exertional angina.

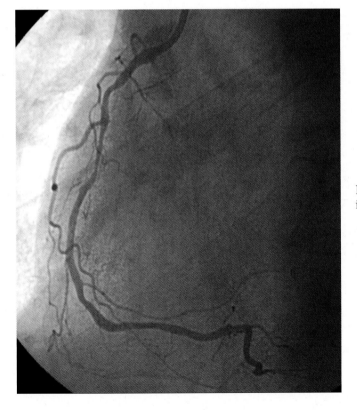

FIGURE 11-6.   Diffuse disease in the right coronary artery involving a long segment of the vessel.

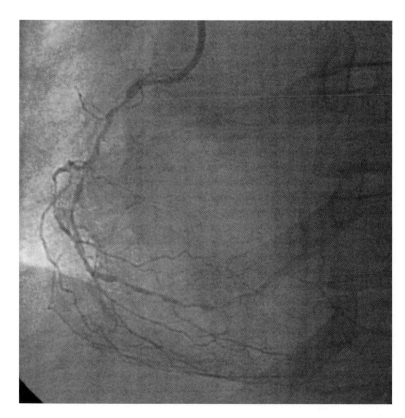

FIGURE 11-7. Obliterative coronary artery disease affecting the right coronary artery in a patient with long-standing diabetes mellitus.

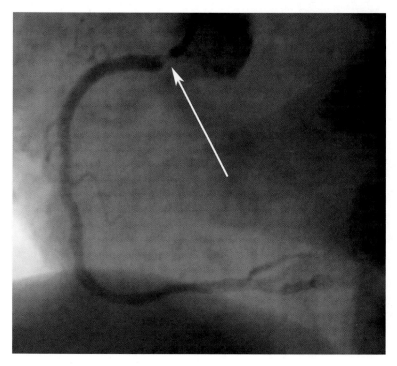

FIGURE 11-8. Severe, ostial stenosis of the right coronary artery.

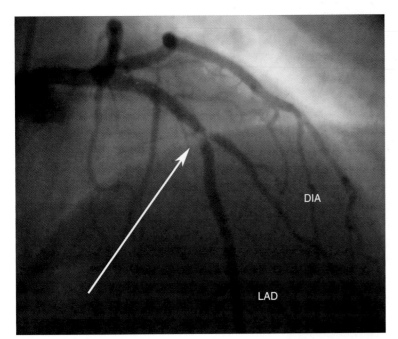

FIGURE 11-9.   Example of a bifurcation steno-sis involving the left anterior descending artery (*LAD*) and a diagonal artery (*DIA*).

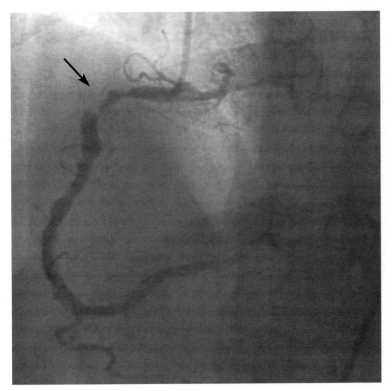

FIGURE 11-10.   This right coronary angiogram was obtained in a patient with an acute coronary syndrome. The lesion in the proximal segment of the artery (*arrow*) is eccentric and irregular.

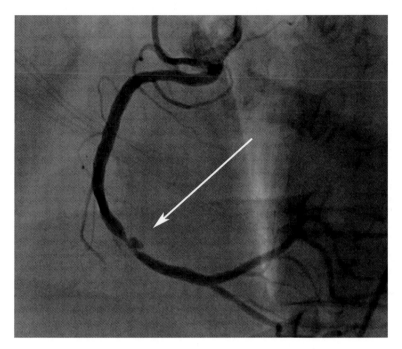

FIGURE 11-11. Ulcerated plaque in the distal right coronary artery *(arrow)* in a patient with a non–ST-segment elevation myocardial infarction.

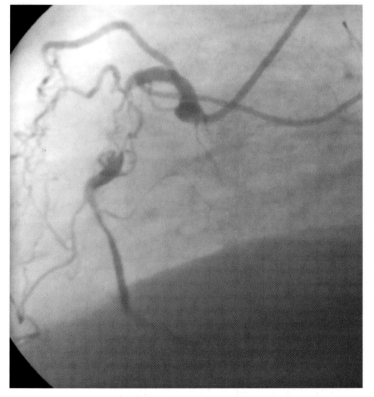

FIGURE 11-12. The right coronary artery is completely occluded in the midportion of the vessel and there are "bridging" collaterals reconstituting the vessel.

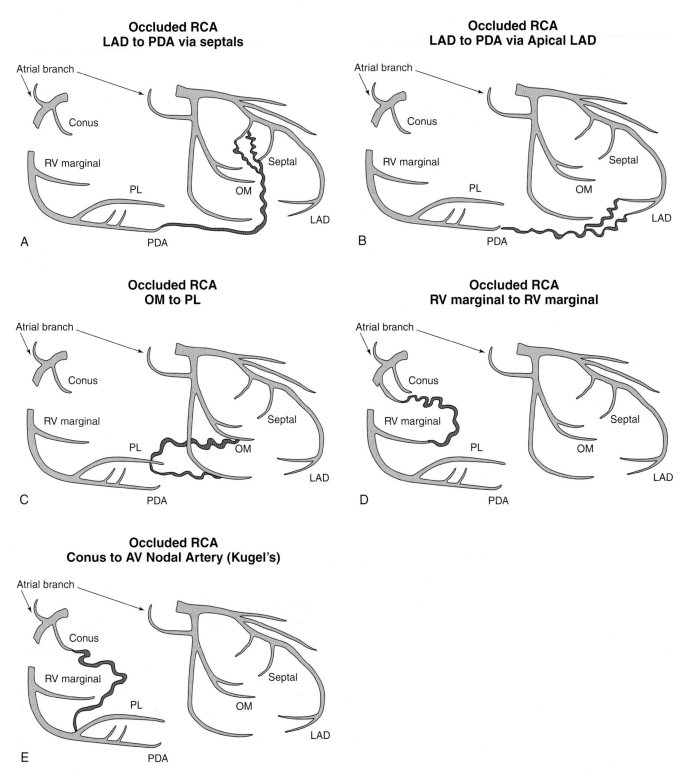

FIGURE 11-13. Commonly observed patterns of collateral formation for an occluded right coronary artery (RCA). (A) LAD to PDA via septals, (B) LAD to PDA via the apical LAD, (C) collateral from OM to PL branch, (D) collateral fro RV marginal proximal to occluded to RV marginal distal, (E) conus to distal RCA via the AV nodal artery. AV, arteriovenous; LAD, left anterior descending artery; OM, obtuse marginal; PDA, posterior descending artery; PL, posterolateral; RV, right ventricular marginal.

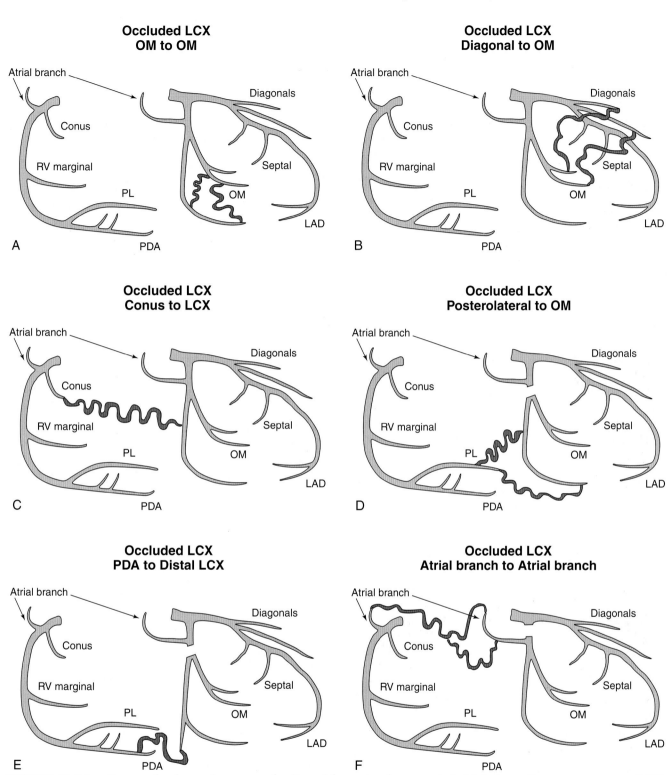

FIGURE 11-14. Commonly observed patterns of collateral formation for an occluded left circumflex coronary artery (LCX) (A) OM to OM collateral, (B) diagnoal to OM collateral, (C) conus branch from RCA to LCX, (D) posterolateral branch from RCA to OM, (E) PDA to distal LCX, (F) atrial branch from right to atrial branch of LCX. LAD, left anterior descending artery; OM, obtuse marginal; PDA, posterior descending artery; PL, posterolateral; RV, right ventricular marginal.

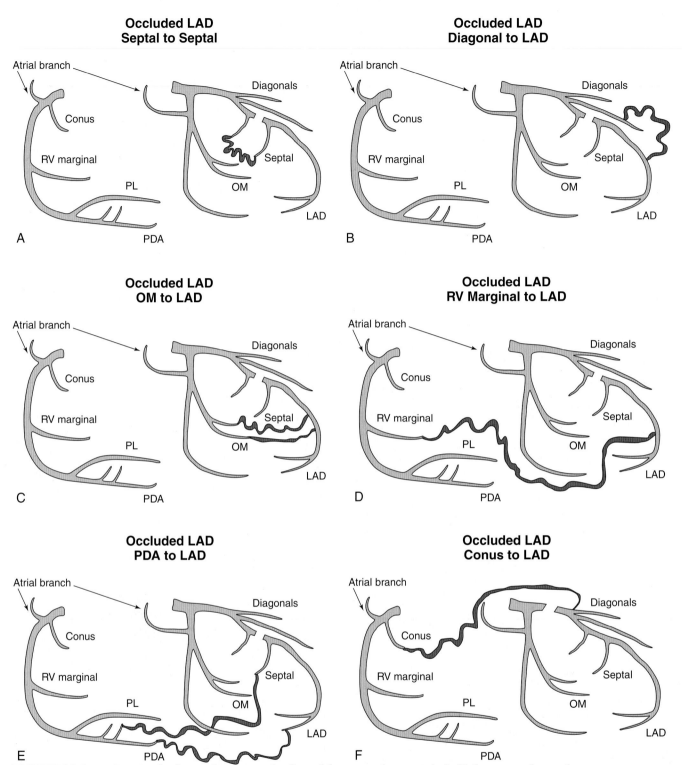

FIGURE 11-15. Commonly observed patterns of collateral formation for an occluded left anterior descending coronary artery. (A) septal to septal collateral, (B) diagonal to distal LAD, (C) OM to LAD, (D) RV marginal to LAD, (E) PDA to LAD, (F) conus branch of RCA to LAD. LAD, left anterior descending artery; OM, obtuse marginal; PDA, posterior descending artery; PL, posterolateral; RV, right ventricular marginal.

CHAPTER 12

ISCHEMIC HEART DISEASE:
BYPASS GRAFT ANGIOGRAPHY

Patients with prior coronary bypass surgery frequently undergo coronary angiography. Selective engagement and imaging of the surgically created conduits may prove challenging to the operator. Furthermore, these vessels are vulnerable to specific pathologic conditions not usually observed in native coronary vessels. Given the huge numbers of patients undergoing coronary bypass operations since the 1980s, this challenging subset will likely form an increasing proportion of coronary angiograms.

Before attempting catheterization, it is essential for the operator to know the anatomic details of the bypass surgery by carefully reviewing the operative report. Failure to do this needlessly exposes the patient to extra radiation and contrast. Many a cardiologist has exhausted themselves and their patients in search of grafts that do not exist or have missed grafts of which they were not aware.

The operative report provides important information regarding the number of proximal anastomoses and whether a single graft provides a conduit to several distal vessels (known as a "jump" or "skip" graft). The operative report also comments on the origin of the graft; saphenous vein conduits may occasionally be attached to unusual locations on the aorta at sites not routinely interrogated by the angiographer. Although most internal mammary grafts are taken in situ from the subclavian artery, the surgeon occasionally uses the internal mammary graft as a "free" graft with the proximal portion of the artery surgically joined to the ascending aorta similar to saphenous veins.

Similar to native coronary angiography, bypass graft angiography requires selective engagement and visualization in several orthogonal views. Care should be taken to image the origin of the graft, the distal anastomosis to the native artery, the body of the graft, and the extent of the native vessel beyond the graft insertion. If all the grafts are not convincingly observed, an aortogram may be necessary to identify the location of a saphenous vein graft or to confirm its occlusion. At the completion of the study, the operator should carefully review the native and graft coronary anatomy to be sure all vascular territories are accounted for.

Saphenous Vein Graft Angiography. Selective engagement of aortosaphenous vein grafts can be challenging. Surgeons sometimes place graft markers on the aorta near the origin of the aortic anastomosis, but this is frequently not done. Figure 12-1 shows the usual location for three commonly used saphenous vein grafts as seen in the left anterior oblique projection. Engagement of vein grafts is often done in the left anterior oblique view with a right Judkins catheter (Fig. 12-2A); the right anterior oblique (RAO) projection tends to better display the proximal origin of the left side grafts (see Fig. 12-2B). Typically, the operator begins the search for unmarked grafts above the native right coronary artery, slowly withdrawing the catheter and turning it slightly clockwise until it "catches" on a graft.

The right coronary artery bypass graft is typically the lowest graft, lying directly above and in the same general orientation as the native right coronary artery. Saphenous vein grafts to the left anterior descending or diagonal branches are usually anastomosed to the aorta above the right graft and in an anterior location on the aorta. Thus, in the left anterior oblique projection, the catheter tip points toward the operator or slightly to the operator's right (see Fig. 12-2A). Saphenous vein grafts to the obtuse marginal arteries are often placed highest on the aorta and are also directed to the operator's right in the left anterior oblique projection.

A variety of catheters may be used to engage saphenous vein grafts. Many can be successfully engaged with a right Judkins catheter. The Amplatz curves (particularly the AR-2) are often used when a right Judkins catheter proves unsuccessful. The proximal segment of a saphenous vein graft to the right coronary artery sharply angles inferiorly, whereas the right Judkins catheter has a tendency to point superiorly in the opposite direction. When a right Judkins catheter does not lie coaxial to the graft and fails to properly opacify a right coronary vein graft adequately, a right bypass catheter is often an improvement. Left bypass catheters are also available and may occasionally help when the right Judkins or Amplatz catheters fail to selectively engage a left-sided graft.

A variety of views can be used to image bypass grafts. In general, it is important to image the origin of the graft, the body of the graft, the distal anastomosis, and the native vessel in two orthogonal views. The views that best image the target vessel are usually chosen (Table 12-1).

Surgeons sometimes use a single saphenous vein graft anastomosed to the aorta to bypass two or more distal target arteries. These sequential grafts are also known as "skip" or "jump" grafts and usually are anastomosed in a side-to-side fashion to one vessel, then continue to terminate in an end-to-side anastomosis. Multiple combinations have been used. Commonly used sequences include a graft to the diagonal that then jumps to an obtuse marginal or a graft to a first obtuse marginal that then jumps to a second obtuse marginal. When performing angiography on sequential grafts, it is important to be sure that each distal anastomosis is well imaged.

Rarely, vein grafts are anastomosed to unusual sites such as the descending aorta (Video 12-1), to an internal mammary artery (IMA; Video 12-2), or at a location very high in the aorta providing

Table 12-1.	Angiographic Projections for Imaging Bypass Grafts

Grafts to Posterior Descending Artery

40 degrees left anterior oblique, 20 degrees cranial

Straight anteroposterior, 20 degrees cranial

30–40 degrees right anterior oblique

Grafts to Obtuse Marginal Artery

40 degrees left anterior oblique

Straight anteroposterior

25 degrees right anterior oblique, 15–20 degrees caudal

Grafts to Diagonal Branches

15 degrees right anterior oblique, 20–30 degrees cranial

40 degrees left anterior oblique, 20 degrees cranial

Grafts to Left Anterior Descending Artery

90 degrees left lateral

15–20 degrees right anterior oblique, 20–30 degrees cranial

40–50 degrees left anterior oblique, 20–30 degrees cranial

25 degrees right anterior oblique, 15–20 degrees caudal

great difficulty with selective engagement particularly if this information is not known to the operator. The case shown in Video 12-1 is such an example and also underscores the importance of reviewing the operative note. This patient had a first bypass operation in 1988 consisting of a right internal mammary graft to the left anterior descending artery and a saphenous vein graft placed to the circumflex with the aortic origin noted by a graft marker. The circumflex vein graft closed, and a second bypass operation performed in 1997 consisting of a saphenous vein graft to the circumflex anastomosed to the descending aorta. Without this knowledge, it is highly unlikely that the circumflex graft would have been found at catheterization and might have been wrongly assumed occluded.

Internal Mammary Graft Angiography. Engagement of the left or right IMAs requires knowledge of the anatomy of the great vessels (Fig. 12-3) and may present technical challenges to the operator. Variations of this anatomy are commonly encountered. For example, the left carotid may originate from the innominate artery instead of the aorta (sometimes called a *bovine* arch), or the left vertebral artery may originate directly from the aorta rather than from the subclavian artery.

A commonly used technique to selectively engage the left IMA is depicted in Figures 12-4 through 12-8. First, a right Judkins catheter is placed in the ascending aorta (see Fig. 12-4). The catheter is gently turned *counterclockwise* and slowly withdrawn until the tip of the catheter points superiorly and into the left subclavian artery (see Fig. 12-5). A few milliliters of contrast is injected to confirm the location of the catheter tip. The catheter is then disconnected from the manifold, and an exchange length, J-tipped, 0.035-inch guide wire is advanced and positioned distally in the subclavian artery (see Fig. 12-6). With the J-wire maintained in this position, the right Judkins catheter is removed and exchanged for an IMA catheter. This catheter is advanced on the guide wire until the tip of this catheter enters the subclavian artery about halfway to the end of the clavicle (see Fig. 12-7). The wire is removed and the catheter is aspirated, flushed, and reattached to the manifold. Another small injection of contrast may be helpful to identify the location of the internal mammary artery. The left internal mammary artery is then selectively engaged by slowly withdrawing the catheter and gently rotating the catheter *counterclockwise*. When the operator believes the catheter is engaged, the catheter tip pressure waveform is examined to be sure there is no damping, which might indicate engagement in the smaller, adjacent branches of the subclavian, or that there is spasm of the IMA. A small injection of contrast confirms engagement and selective angiography of the IMA is performed (see Fig. 12-8). Commonly used angiographic views include the straight anteroposterior projection, an RAO cranial projection, and the lateral projection. The anastomosis may be more clearly seen in the RAO caudal projection.

Alternative techniques to engage the left IMA are sometimes used. For example, some operators place the IMA catheter in the descending aorta and try to pass a hydrophilic glide wire into the subclavian artery by making multiple passes from this position and then advancing the catheter directly into the subclavian.

In patients with left internal mammary grafts, it is important to screen for the presence of a subclavian stenosis proximal to the origin of the internal mammary (Video 12-3). All patients undergoing catheterization with an in situ left internal mammary graft should, at minimum, have blood pressure measured in both arms and a careful physical examination for subclavian bruits. Angiography of the subclavian should be performed and a pressure measurement made across the subclavian stenosis in the presence of suspected subclavian stenosis. In general, in the presence of an internal mammary graft, a pressure gradient of at least 10 to 20 mm Hg is believed to represent a significant stenosis.

In addition to the presence of subclavian stenosis, severe tortuosity of the aorta and/or subclavian artery proximal to the IMA may create great difficulties for the operator. Selective engagement of the IMA may not be possible in such cases (Video 12-4). A long (80-cm) sheath may help by straightening some of the iliac and aortic tortuosity, but if most of the difficulty lies with subclavian tortuosity, then it may remain impossible to engage the left internal mammary from the femoral access. If this is encountered, and if it remains important to image the internal mammary graft, then a left brachial approach is required.

It is important to use great care when manipulating the IMA catheter in the subclavian; dissection of the subclavian artery and IMA may occur and lead to closure of the graft (Video 12-5).

Surgeons may use the right IMA to graft the posterior descending artery or a branch of the circumflex system; in some circumstances, this conduit may also be used to graft the left anterior descending artery (Video 12-6). The technique used to engage the right IMA is similar to the one described for the left internal mammary by first engaging the innominate artery with a right Judkins catheter followed by an exchange for the IMA catheter.

Other Coronary Bypass Conduits. The right gastroepiploic artery has been used by surgeons as a conduit to bypass lesions in the right coronary artery. The gastroepiploic artery is a branch of the hepatic artery, which, in turn, is a branch of the celiac trunk (Fig. 12-9). Selective angiography of this vessel is performed in the lateral projection using a right Judkins catheter, an IMA catheter, or a Cobra angiographic catheter. Radial artery grafts are anastomosed to the aorta at locations similar to saphenous veins; the techniques used to engage these grafts are the same as those used for saphenous veins. Radial artery grafts usually appear smaller than vein grafts and are prone to spasm. Rarely, an artificial or prosthetic conduit is used to bypass the coronary arteries. The Cabrol procedure is typically performed in patients with proximal aortic dissection, and aortic valve and cusp involvement. The proximal aorta is replaced with a large (25–30-mm diameter) tubular prosthesis outfitted with a prosthetic valve. Another, smaller (8-mm) tube graft is anastomosed in a side-to-side fashion to the aortic conduit, and each distal end of this tube graft is used to bypass the right and left main coronary arteries. Angiography of this large conduit is usually simple. A right Judkins catheter is often used, and imaging of the conduit provides angiography of the entire coronary circulation (Videos 12-7 and 12-8).

Bypass Graft Pathology. The saphenous veins and arterial conduits used for bypass surgery are subject to occlusion and narrowing. Approximately 10% of vein grafts occlude early after surgery, and up to 15% to 20% are closed after 1 year. The vein graft attrition rate is roughly 1% to 2% per year for the first 5 years and about 4% per year after this. Thus, by 10 years, more than 50% of vein grafts are occluded. The left internal mammary graft has a much better patency rate; more than 90% of these grafts remain patent 10 years after surgery. The natural history of other arterial grafts or free left internal mammary arterial grafts is less well known, but patency rates are likely intermediate between those observed for saphenous vein and in situ left IMA grafts.

The pathology of graft disease varies depending on the time from surgery. Early occlusion is typically thrombotic and caused by technical problems at the time of surgery, poor quality of the vein graft, or the presence of diffuse disease in the target vessel with poor runoff. Lesions occurring at the aorto-ostial or distal anastomosis seen in the first year after surgery usually represent intimal proliferation (Video 12-9). Disease found in the body of a vein graft is usually due to atheromatous degeneration and is observed in vein grafts older than 3 years (Video 12-10). Severe atherosclerotic changes in old vein grafts lead to diffuse narrowing and filling defects ("degenerated" vein grafts) (Videos 12-11 and 12-12). Pathologic examination of these grafts reveals bulky, friable atheroma, and percutaneous intervention of these lesions is associated with a very high risk for distal embolization.

The IMA is generally believed to be highly resistant to atherosclerosis. Lesions of the body of the IMA are unusual. Rarely, lesions may be seen at the origin of the internal mammary from the subclavian artery and represent either atherosclerosis originating in the subclavian artery or catheter-induced arterial injury and intimal proliferation from prior catheter engagements (Fig. 12-10). Distal anastomotic lesions may also occur, likely from intimal proliferation at the target vessel site (Video 12-13). The IMA may also become atretic or occluded if it is used to graft an artery that is not stenotic or if it is mishandled during surgery (Videos 12-14 and 12-15).

Unusual angiographic findings in patients with prior bypass surgery include fistulous connections between the vein graft and a coronary vein (Video 12-16), saphenous vein aneurysms (Videos 12-17 and 12-18), and aneurysm at the graft-native vessel anastomosis (Video 12-19).

Suggested Readings

1. Motwani JG, Topol EJ: Aortocoronary saphenous vein graft disease. Pathogenesis, predisposition, and prevention. Circulation 1998;97:916–931.
2. Gelsomino S, Frassani R, Da Col P, et al: A long-term experience with the Cabrol root replacement technique for the management of ascending aortic aneurysms and dissections. Ann Thorac Surg 2003;75:126–131.

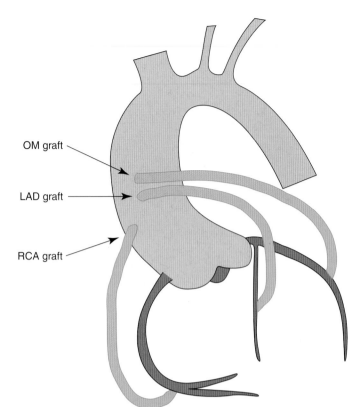

FIGURE 12-1. Cartoon demonstrating the usual placement of the saphenous vein grafts on the aorta in the left anterior oblique projection. LAD, left anterior descending; OM, obtuse marginal; RCA, right coronary artery.

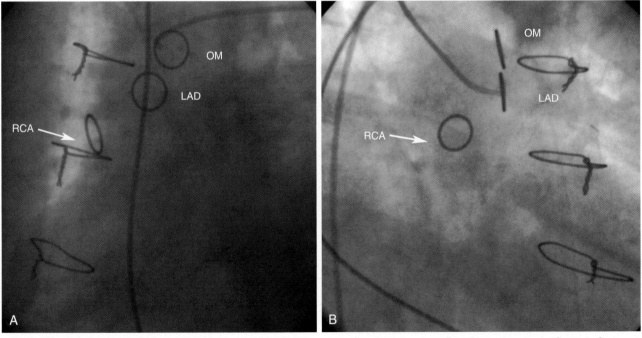

FIGURE 12-2. Example of surgical markers placed on the aorta to localize the site of saphenous vein graft. *A,* Left anterior oblique projection. *B,* Right anterior oblique projection. LAD, left anterior descending; OM, obtuse marginal; RCA, right coronary artery.

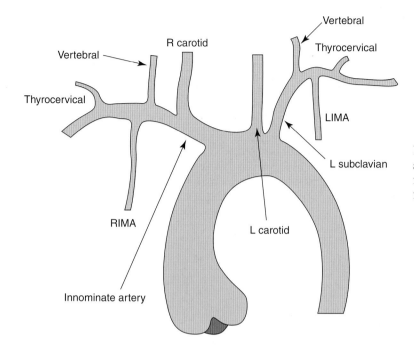

FIGURE 12-3. Diagram of the arch of the aorta and its major branches. L, left; LIMA, left internal mammary artery; R, right; RIMA, right internal mammary artery.

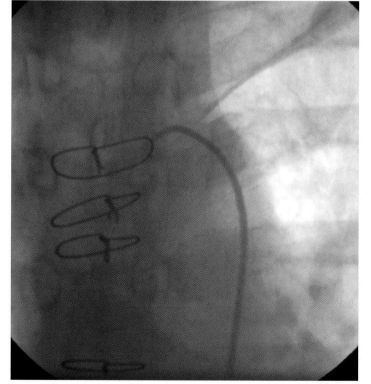

FIGURE 12-4. Technique to engage the left internal mammary artery from femoral access. Step 1: A right Judkins catheter is positioned in the aorta between the innominate artery and left subclavian artery.

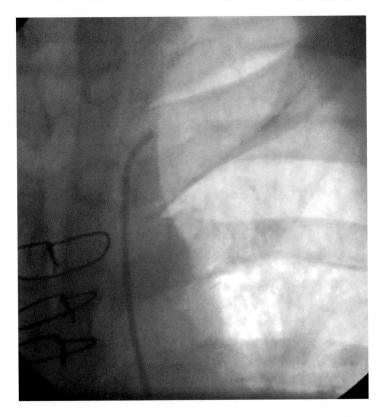

FIGURE 12-5. Technique to engage the left internal mammary artery from femoral access. Step 2: The right Judkins catheter is turned counterclockwise until the tip points into the left subclavian artery. At this point, a small amount of contrast can be injected to confirm the position of the catheter.

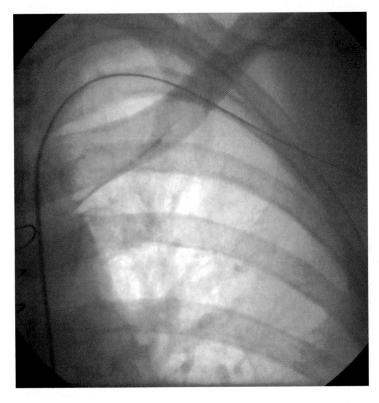

FIGURE 12-6. Technique to engage the left internal mammary artery from femoral access. Step 3: An exchange length, 0.035-inch guide wire is positioned into the left subclavian artery via the right Judkins catheter, and the right Judkins catheter is removed and replaced with an internal mammary (IMA) catheter.

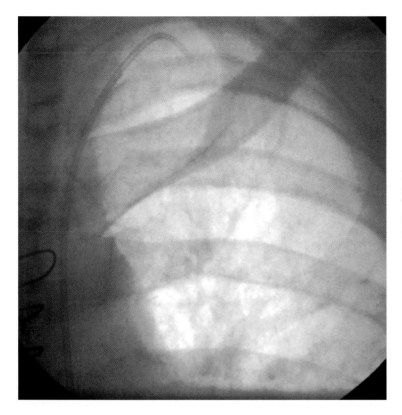

FIGURE 12-7. Technique to engage the left internal mammary artery (IMA) from femoral access. Step 4: The IMA catheter is slowly drawn back and gently turned counterclockwise to engage the left internal mammary artery.

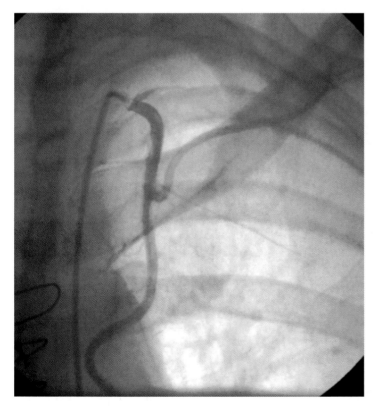

FIGURE 12-8. Technique to engage the left internal mammary artery from femoral access. Step 5: The left internal mammary is selective engaged and angiography is performed.

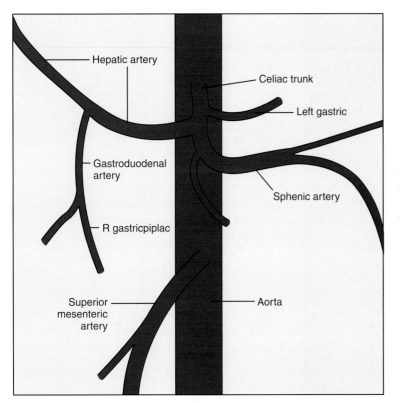

FIGURE 12-9. The gastroepiploic artery is a branch of the gastroduodenal artery that branches from the common hepatic artery, which, in turn, is a branch of the celiac trunk.

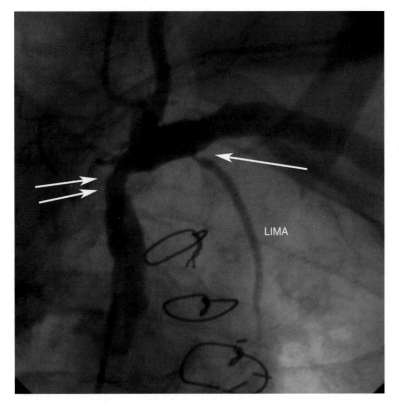

FIGURE 12-10. Atherosclerotic disease of the left internal mammary artery is rare. In this case, there is severe narrowing of the ostium of the left internal mammary artery that was used to graft the left anterior descending artery (*arrow*). This graft had been previously instrumented several times in the past during prior cardiac catheterizations and previously appeared normal. Atherosclerotic disease of the subclavian artery proximal to the left internal mammary artery (*LIMA; double arrow*) also is present.

CHAPTER 13

ADVANCED CORONARY ANGIOGRAPHY

Several conditions commonly encountered during coronary angiography lead to technical challenges or diagnostic quandaries. These include marked vessel tortuosity, coronary artery calcification, ectasia, aneurysm, thrombus, and spasm. The experienced operator should be aware of the common imaging artifacts potentially causing interpretation errors and mismanagement, and be prepared to occasionally stumble upon unexpected findings or rare conditions.

Vessel Tortuosity. Marked tortuosity of the coronary arteries may occur in elderly patients and in those with long-standing hypertension. As a consequence of excessive vessel tortuosity, several coronary segments may be obscured from overlapping vessels or foreshortening artifact (Fig. 13-1 and Video 13-1). Lesions within these locations may be missed or erroneously interpreted. Optimal imaging requires multiple views with unusual angulation. When excessive tortuosity is present, the angiographer should carefully review the angiogram to be sure that each segment is clearly seen before completing the case.

Coronary Artery Calcification. Coronary calcification is a common finding on angiography. Calcification appears as a linear, dense opacification outlining one or more of the coronary arteries (Video 13-2). Extensive calcification of the coronary can create the appearance of a filling defect leading to its misinterpretation as a thrombus (Videos 13-3 and 13-4). Angiography cannot determine whether calcification is superficial and involves the atherosclerotic plaque or whether it is confined to deeper layers of the arterial wall sparing the plaque. This can best be learned by intravascular ultrasound.

Coronary Ectasia and Aneurysm. Coronary artery aneurysms are usually defined as an area of abnormal dilatation greater than 1.5 times an adjacent normal reference segment (Fig. 13-2). They are relatively rare findings observed in 1.5% to 5.0% of patients undergoing angiography, and are more common in the right coronary artery than the other epicardial arteries (1, 2). Involvement of the left main coronary is rare. There are many potential causes of coronary artery aneurysms (Table 13-1). The most common cause (50% of cases) is atherosclerosis. Kawasaki disease is the second most common cause. Aneurysms may rarely develop after a percutaneous coronary intervention. Some of these may represent a "pseudoaneurysm" from a contained perforation at the time of the intervention. The other causes are rare.

Although many coronary aneurysms are found incidentally at the time of angiography, some may be responsible for the presenting syndrome (Video 13-5). When symptomatic, they may lead to ischemia either from a coexisting stenosis involving the aneurysmal segment or from abnormal flow patterns leading to in situ thrombus formation and distal embolization. Rupture of large coronary artery aneurysms has been reported but is rare. Similarly, large aneurysms may cause symptoms from compression of adjacent cardiac chambers, but this is

Table 13-1.	Causes of Coronary Artery Aneurysms

Atherosclerosis

Congenital conditions

Post-traumatic causes

Postpercutaneous coronary intervention

Connective tissue diseases
  Marfan syndrome
  Ehlers–Danlos syndrome

Inflammatory causes
  Kawasaki disease
  Takayasu arteritis
  Rheumatoid arthritis
  Polyarteritis nodosa

Infection
  Syphilis
  Bacterial endocarditis

also a rare sequela of a coronary artery aneurysm. Prognosis is related to the degree and severity of underlying atherosclerosis. Large aneurysms associated with a significant stenosis or symptoms, or both, are treated surgically or with covered stents. Treatment of asymptomatic coronary artery aneurysms without underlying stenosis is controversial. Anticoagulation therapy with both antiplatelet drugs and warfarin is often prescribed but is based on anecdotal experience. Because rupture is rare, prophylactic surgery for coronary artery aneurysms is not usually warranted. Examples of a variety of atherosclerotic aneurysms are shown in Videos 13-6 through 13-9.

An example of a coronary artery aneurysm from Kawasaki disease (or mucocutaneous lymph node syndrome) is shown in Video 13-10. This vasculitis usually affects infants and small children manifesting as fever, skin rash, lymphadenopathy, conjunctivitis, and mucosal changes. Coronary artery involvement is its most important sequela, present in about 20% of cases. Rarely (<1% of cases), other vessels such as the brachial, renal, mesenteric, and iliac arteries may be involved. Coronary aneurysms can cause myocardial infarction and sudden death. Over time, the aneurysms regress in about 50% of cases.

Coronary Thrombus. Many patients with acute coronary syndromes (unstable angina or acute myocardial infarction) undergo coronary angiography as part of an invasive management strategy. These syndromes are usually caused by rupture of a vulnerable plaque culminating in the development of an occlusive thrombus.

Angiographically, thrombus is diagnosed when a discrete, intraluminal filling defect outlined by contrast with clearly defined borders is observed within the arterial lumen (Fig. 13-3). Persistent contrast staining may or may not be present. Other angiographic features suggesting but less diagnostic of a thrombus include a filling defect without well-defined borders or the presence of haziness, representing diminished contrast density, within a segment of the artery. These later findings are not specific for thrombus and may be seen in eccentric plaque without thrombus or from severe vessel wall calcification. In patients with acute coronary syndromes, thrombi often dangle from the distal end of a severe stenosis (Videos 13-11 through 13-13). Thrombi evident by angiography are usually large; smaller clots escape detection by this technique. Coronary angioscopy, primarily a research tool, is a much more sensitive technique for diagnosing intraluminal clot (3–5).

Not all coronary thrombi originate within the vessel; some represent embolism. The absence of atherosclerotic disease at the site of a filling defect suggests an embolism. An additional clue relates to the location of the intraluminal defect. Coronary emboli often lodge at branch points in the artery. At these sites, the vessel lumen diameter tapers substantially, thereby trapping an embolism. Coronary emboli may represent clot originating from a cardiac chamber or structure. For example, an embolism may arise from the left ventricle in a patient after myocardial infarction, the left atrium in a patient with atrial fibrillation, or from a left-sided valve in a patient with thrombosis of a mechanical valve. Emboli may also arise from vegetation in an individual with endocarditis.

Coronary Artery Spasm. In the cardiac catheterization laboratory, coronary spasm is commonly provoked by catheters during selective coronary engagement or from instrumentation of the artery with equipment used to perform a coronary interventional procedure. Syndromes of spontaneous coronary spasm (i.e., Prinzmetal's angina) may rarely be serendipitously observed during cardiac catheterization in patients under evaluation for chest pain.

Catheter-related coronary spasm is frequently encountered and does not imply an underlying tendency for spontaneous spasm. It is especially common in the right coronary artery, particularly in young persons with normal vessels (Videos 13-14 and 13-15). Catheter-induced spasm of the left main artery is rare; however, a catheter may provoke spasm of the proximal left anterior descending artery or the left circumflex in the event of subselective engagement of these vessels (Videos 13-16 and 13-17). Often, the spasm develops as soon as the catheter is engaged, causing pressure damping and ventricularization. Catheter tip spasm is often misinterpreted as an atherosclerotic ostial lesion. Clues to the presence of catheter tip spasm include the lack of atherosclerosis at any other location, fluctuating appearance of the lesion, and any lesion located at the very tip of a diagnostic catheter, particularly in the right coronary artery. When catheter spasm is suspected, nitroglycerine (administered either sublingually or directly into the artery) restores the arterial lumen to normal, confirming the diagnosis. Spasm may be intense and prolonged; severe cases may lead to ischemia and significant sequelae such as arrhythmia. In the event of prolonged or refractory spasm, the catheter should be removed and repeated doses of systemic nitroglycerin used. Gentle reengagement of the artery can be attempted after 10 to 15 minutes.

Coronary spasm is frequently encountered during an interventional procedure. Any aspect of coronary instrumentation including insertion of a guide catheter, placement of a guide wire, and advancement of any device (balloon, stent catheters, rotational or directional atherectomy, and intravascular ultrasound catheters) can cause spasm. Unrecognized spasm during an intervention may be misdiagnosed as a complication such as dissection or plaque shift and improperly managed.

Cocaine is a well-known cause of coronary vasospasm; spasm may occur days to weeks after ingestion (Videos 13-18 and 13-19). Spontaneous coronary vasospasm, or Prinzmetal's angina, is relatively uncommon. In the classic case, a patient has ischemic rest chest pain with ST-segment elevation, followed by resolution of the pain and ST-segment elevation with nitroglycerin. Episodes may occur at rest or relate to exertion. It has been associated with smoking, Raynaud's phenomenon, migraine headache, hyperventilation, and cold stimulation. The diagnosis is usually made purely on clinical grounds and is typically made when ischemic chest pain at rest is observed with ST-segment elevation with an angiogram showing normal coronary arteries. Although classically described with angiographic normal arteries, spontaneous coronary spasm may occur in the setting of varying degrees of atherosclerotic narrowing (Videos 13-20 and 13-21).

Rarely, the diagnosis is made in the cardiac catheterization laboratory when the patient fortuitously experiences development of symptoms and ST-segment elevation during the procedure. The typical angiographic appearance is a focal segmental narrowing with a smooth, tapered appearance (Videos 13-22 and 13-23). Although provocative testing with ergonovine, acetylcholine, and hyperventilation have been described, their specificity is low; most clinicians find them to be of little value.

Angiographic Artifacts. It is important for an angiographer to distinguish a pathologic finding from an artifact. Many potential artifacts lead to erroneous image interpretation. Poor injection technique causes contrast streaming and inadequate opacification, potentially obscuring lesions or leading the angiographer to falsely interpret the presence of a dissection flap or a filling defect. Competitive flow from collateral vessels or bypass grafts is sometimes misinterpreted as intracoronary thrombus or an eccentric lesion (Video 13-24). Similarly, the swirling of contrast that sometimes occurs in the presence of large, patulous arteries or saphenous vein grafts may mislead the operator to diagnose thrombus or atheromatous disease. Small, overlying vessels may be misconstrued as a lesion or a dissection. Vessel foreshortening may cause a lesion to narrow the lumen more than it actually does.

A common artifact seen during a coronary intervention is due to the straightening of a tortuous segment of a coronary artery by a stiff guide wire. This "pseudolesion" is due to invagination of the redundant artery at the site of vessel tortuosity and has a characteristic appearance (Fig. 13-4). Although most cases of straightening artifact demonstrate this typical appearance, occasionally it can be difficult to determine whether an abnormal angiographic finding occurring in this setting represents straightening artifact or another problem such as arterial dissection.

Other Unusual Findings on Coronary Angiography. Several rare findings have been observed on coronary angiography. Recanalized total occlusions have a peculiar "dual-lumen" or a beaded appearance (Videos 13-25 and 13-26). This finding is often misinterpreted as a thrombus. Spontaneous coronary dissection is a rare condition largely affecting young women during or after pregnancy and patients with connective tissue diseases (6). The entity may present as an acute coronary syndrome with angiography revealing intimal flaps within one or more of the coronary arteries (Videos 13-27 and 13-28).

Cardiac tumors are rare. Coronary angiography sometimes displays the blood supply to the tumor known as a "tumor blush" (Videos 13-29 through 13-31). These are unusual findings. Despite the presence of a large tumor, some myxomas do not have a demonstrable blood supply by angiography (Video 13-32).

References

1. Wang KY, Ting CT, Sutton MS, Chen YT: Coronary artery aneurysms: A 25-patient study. Catheter Cardiovasc Interv 1999;48:31–38.
2. Syed M, Lesch M: Coronary artery aneurysms. A review. Prog Cardiovasc Dis 1997;40:77–84.
3. Teirstein PS, Schatz RA, DeNardo SJ, et al: Angioscopic versus angiographic detection of thrombus during coronary interventional procedures. Am J Cardiol 1995;75:1083–1087.
4. Uretsky BF, Denys BG, Counihan PC, Ragosta M: Angioscopic evaluation of incompletely obstructing coronary intraluminal filling defects: Comparison to angiography. Cathet Cardiovasc Diagn 1994;33:323–329.
5. White CJ, Ramee SR, Collins TJ, et al: Coronary thrombi increase PTCA risk: Angioscopy as a clinical tool. Circulation 1996;93:253–258.
6. Almeda FQ, Barkatullah S, Kavinsky CJ: Spontaneous coronary artery dissection. Clin Cardiol 2004;27:377–380.

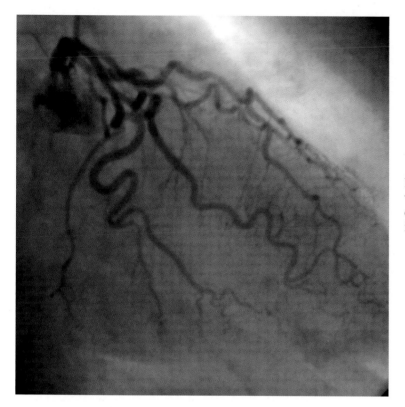

FIGURE 13-1. Marked vessel tortuosity in a patient with long-standing hypertension. In such cases, it is difficult to adequately image all coronary segments free of overlapping vessels.

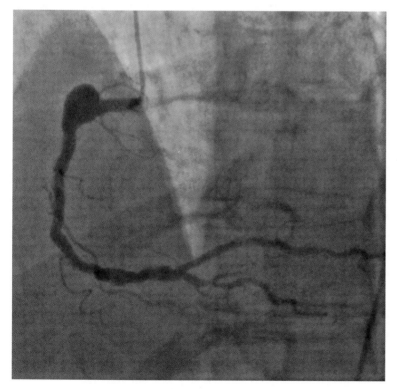

FIGURE 13-2. Left anterior oblique projection of the right coronary artery in a patient with a large aneurysm involving the proximal segment of the artery.

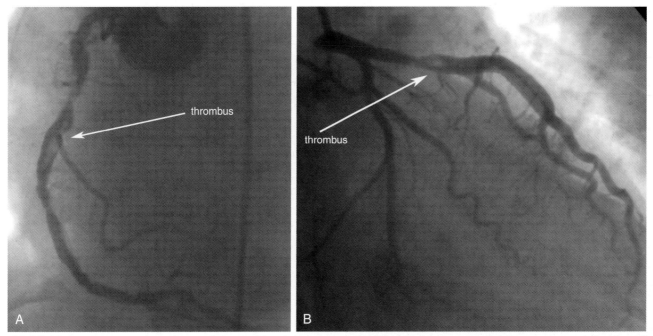

FIGURE 13-3.   Coronary thrombus is diagnosed by the presence of a filling defect surrounded by contrast on all sides. The clot often hangs from the distal end of a severely narrowed atherosclerotic segment (*A*) but may also appear distal to a lesion of lesser severity (*B*).

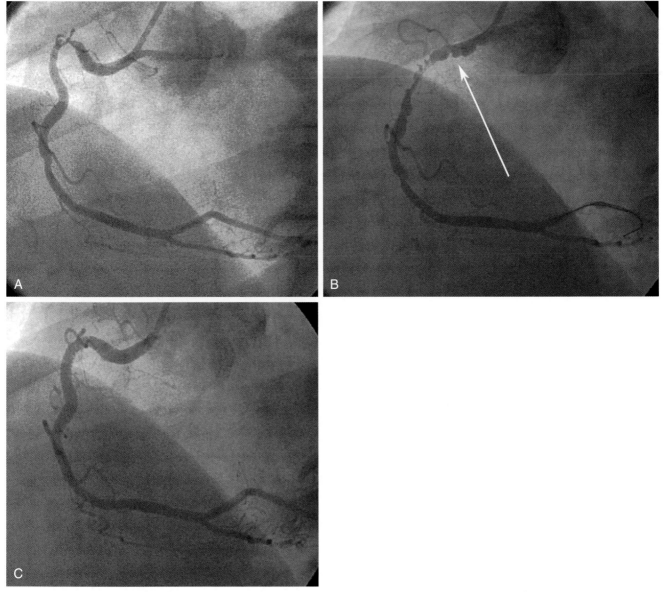

FIGURE 13-4. During coronary intervention, a guide wire placed down a coronary artery may artificially straighten the artery and create an angiographic artifact known as a pseudolesion. *A,* The proximal segment of the right coronary artery is angulated with a severe stenosis just distal to the bend. After an angioplasty guide wire was placed, the artery straightened and created the appearance of a lesion within the previously angled segment *(B, arrow).* The smooth appearance represents invagination of the artery. This "lesion" disappeared when the guide wire was removed at the end of the procedure *(C).*

CHAPTER 14

CORONARY ANOMALIES

The coronary arteries consistently originate from the same location on the aorta, following a similar and predictable course on the surface of the heart facilitating the performance and interpretation of coronary angiography. Occasionally, one or more of the coronary arteries cannot be found in its customary origin on the aorta, or the artery may originate normally but branch, terminate, or distribute itself in a highly unusual manner. These variations from the normal anatomy are known as *coronary anomalies*.

By definition, coronary anomalies are rare. Among patients undergoing coronary angiography, the incidence depends on the population studied and the criteria used to define an anomaly. One large study reported an incidence rate of coronary anomalies of 1.3% for adults undergoing catheterization primarily for the detection of coronary artery disease (1). Anomalous coronary arteries can be defined based on the relative frequency of anatomic variations in the general population (2). Normal anatomy describes any morphologic feature observed in more than 1% of an unselected population, whereas the term *normal variant* describes an alternative, relatively unusual morphologic feature but still seen in more than 1% of the same population. An anomaly, therefore, would be defined as a morphologic feature identified in less than 1% of the population.

Most anomalous coronary arteries discovered by angiography represent interesting curiosities and have no clinical significance. However, some specific anomalies have the potential for serious sequelae and some may cause cardiac symptoms or events including chest pain, syncope, heart failure, dyspnea, ventricular arrhythmia, myocardial infarction, and sudden death.

The potential clinical consequences of coronary anomalies are summarized in Table 14-1. If an artery is not visualized and the anomaly unnoticed, the operator may misinterpret this finding as an occluded vessel, or the operator may misidentify an anomalous vessel, mistaking it for another artery. Similarly, if the anomalous vessel is not visualized, significant coronary disease may be present in that vessel and go undetected. Several coronary anomalies, specifically large coronary fistulae, anomalous origin of the left coronary artery coursing between the pulmonary artery and the aorta, and perhaps myocardial bridges, may result in episodic ischemia, usually after extreme exertion. The mechanism by which some of these coronary anomalies cause myocardial ischemia is not clearly established. It is believed that patients with anomalous origin of a coronary artery from the pulmonary artery and patients with large fistulae develop coronary steal or intercoronary shunting as the responsible mechanism. Anomalous origin from a contralateral coronary sinus is associated with acute angulation of the proximal artery or a "slitlike" orifice compromising the lumen and causing ischemia. Finally, anomalous vessels coursing between the aorta and the pulmonary artery are thought to be subject to compression of the artery particularly during exertion. Several coronary anomalies are important to recognize before heart surgery to avoid injury of these vessels during the procedure. Coronaries with aberrant or ectopic origins may prove technically difficult to perform percutaneous interventions because of difficulty with guide catheter placement and

Table 14-1.	Potential Clinical Consequences of Specific Coronary Anomalies

Myocardial Ischemia

1. Fistula
2. Anomalous left coronary artery from PA
3. Anomalous origin from AO
4. Myocardial bridge

Endocarditis

1. Fistula

Volume Overload

1. Fistula
2. Anomalous left coronary artery from PA

Cardiomyopathy

1. Anomalous left coronary artery from PA

Complications during Surgery

1. Anomalous origin from AO
2. Myocardial bridge

Technical Difficulties with PCI

1. Anomalous origin from AO

Sudden Cardiac Death

1. Anomalous origin from AO
    a. Left coronary from right sinus coursing between PA and AO
    b. Left coronary from the PA
    c. Right coronary from the left sinus coursing between PA and AO
    d. Single coronary artery from the right sinus

AO, aorta; PA, pulmonary artery; PCI, percutaneous coronary intervention.

Adapted from Angelini P, Velasco JA, Flamm S: Coronary anomalies: Incidence, pathophysiology, and clinical relevance. Circulation 2002;105:2449–2454, by permission.

backup. Certain rare coronary anomalies have been associated with sudden cardiac death in young athletes and during exercise.

Classification and Incidence of Specific Coronary Anomalies

An impressive array of coronary anomalies has been described. These anomalies can be classified as follows: (a) anomalies of coronary artery origin and course, (b) anomalies of the intrinsic coronary anatomy, and (c) anomalies of coronary termination (Table 14-2). The overall and relative frequencies of these coronary anomalies obtained from a large (126,595 patients) angiographic study are shown in Table 14-3 (1). Six specific anomalies account for nearly 90% of the observed anomalies; the remainder are rare.

Several congenital heart defects are associated with anomalies of the coronary arteries. Bicuspid aortic valves and coarctation of the aorta are associated with absence of the left main (also called a *split* left main) where the left circumflex and left anterior descending arteries each originate separately from the aorta. Complete transposition of the great arteries is associated with the following anomalies: (a) left circumflex from the right coronary artery, (b) single coronary artery from either sinus, (c) origin of both arteries from the inappropriate sinuses, and (d) left anterior descending artery originating from the right coronary artery.

Table 14-2.	Classification of Coronary Anomalies

1. Anomalies of Origin and Course

a. Separate ostia of the left circumflex and left anterior descending artery

b. Anomalous location in the root in the proper sinus
    i. High or low origin of the left coronary artery
    ii. High or low origin of the right coronary artery

c. Anomalous origin from a different coronary sinus
    i. Right coronary artery from the left sinus
    ii. Left coronary artery from the right sinus
    iii. Left circumflex from the right sinus
    iv. Left anterior descending from the right sinus
    v. Single coronary artery from either the right or left sinus

d. Anomalous origin from a location other than coronary sinus
    i. Left coronary artery from the pulmonary artery
    ii. Right coronary artery from the pulmonary artery
    iii. Either left or right coronary from descending aorta, ascending aorta, or branches of the aorta

2. Anomalies of Intrinsic Coronary Anatomy

a. Congenital coronary ectasia or aneurysm

b. Absent or hypoplastic coronary artery

c. Myocardial bridge

d. Anomalous distribution
    i. Posterior descending artery from the left anterior descending
    ii. Absent PDA or split right coronary artery
    iii. Absent or split left anterior descending artery
    iv. Ectopic origin of the first septal perforator from right coronary artery

3. Anomalies of Coronary Termination

a. Fistulae from the right coronary or left coronary arteries to:
    i. Pulmonary artery
    ii. Right ventricle
    iii. Coronary (intercoronary communication)
    iv. Right atrium
    v. Coronary sinus
    vi. Superior vena cava
    vii. Pulmonary vein
    viii. Left atrium
    ix. Left ventricle

Corrected transposition of the great arteries is associated with a single coronary artery from the right facing sinus. Tetralogy of Fallot has several associated anomalies. The most common consists of an abnormally long and large conus artery. In 4% to 5% of cases, the left anterior descending artery arises anomalously from the right coronary artery or the right coronary sinus passing across the right ventricular outflow tract. Rarely, other anomalies may be seen including a single coronary artery from either the right or left sinus with a major branch traversing across the right ventricular outflow tract or an anomalous origin of the left circumflex from the right sinus.

Anomalies of Origin and Course

Normal Anatomy. Figure 14-1 demonstrates the normal origins of the coronary arteries from the coronary sinuses, and their proximal course relative to the aorta and the pulmonary

Table 14-3.	Relative Frequency of Specific Coronary Anomalies	
ANOMALY	INCIDENCE (%)	% OF ANOMALIES
Absent left main	0.41	30.4
LCX from RCA	0.37	27.7
Ectopic RCA in right cusp	0.15	11.2
Small fistulae	0.12	9.7
RCA from left cusp	0.11	8.1
Large fistulae	0.05	3.7
LAD from right cusp	0.03	2.3
Left main from right cusp	0.02	1.3
Single coronary	0.02	1.3
Ectopic left main from left cusp	0.013	0.95
Left main from pulmonary artery	0.008	0.59
Absent LCX	0.003	0.24
RCA from noncoronary cusp	0.003	0.24
Intercoronary communication	0.002	0.18
RCA from pulmonary artery	0.002	0.12

LAD, left anterior descending artery; LCX, left circumflex; RCA, right coronary artery.

Adapted from Yamanaka O, Hobbs RE: Coronary artery anomalies in 126,595 patients undergoing coronary arteriography. Cath Cardiovasc Diagn 1990;21:28–40, by permission.

outflow tract. In a right-dominant circulation, the right coronary artery originates from the right sinus of Valsalva, courses within the atrioventricular groove giving off right ventricular marginal branches to the surface of the right ventricle, and continues in the atrioventricular groove to the "crux", where it branches into the posterolateral and the posterior descending arteries. The posterior descending artery lies in the posterior aspect of the interventricular groove supplying septal perforators to the interventricular septum. The left coronary artery originates from the left, or anterior, sinus of Valsalva dividing after a short distance into the left anterior descending and left circumflex arteries. The left anterior descending artery runs along the anterior aspect of the interventricular groove supplying septal perforators to the interventricular septum and diagonal arteries to the lateral wall of the heart. Similar to the right coronary artery, the circumflex artery runs in the atrioventricular groove supplying the obtuse marginal arteries to the lateral surface of the heart. In left-dominant circulations, the circumflex terminates with a posterior descending artery in the posterior interventricular groove, and the right coronary artery terminates in the atrioventricular groove supplying only right ventricular branches.

Specific Anomalies. The anomalies of origin and course can be classified into four subtypes: (a) absence of the left main; (b) anomalous origin of the coronary ostium in the aortic root but in the proper sinus; (c) anomalous origin from a different coronary sinus, and (d) anomalous origin from a location other than a coronary sinus (see Table 14-2).

Absence of the Left Main. Also known as a *split* left main, absence of the left main coronary is one of the most common coronary anomalies. Separate ostia of the circumflex and left anterior descending artery from the left coronary sinus characterize this anomaly (Fig. 14-2; Videos 14-1 and 14-2). Absence of the left main is associated with bicuspid aortic valves and coarctation of the aorta. This entity has no clinical significance except that it may be a source of missed diagnosis or technical difficulty during angiography. In addition, failure to identify this anomaly may lead to the false conclusion that the nonimaged vessel is occluded; or if this anomaly is not appreciated, coronary disease in the nonimaged artery may go undetected. Selective engagement of each of the vessels may pose minor technical challenges. Typically, the standard-length Judkins catheter (JL-4) selectively engages the left anterior descending artery; in such cases, a longer catheter (e.g., a JL-5) successfully engages the circumflex. Alternatively, rotation of the Judkins catheter in a clockwise fashion may selectively engage the circumflex, and a counterclockwise turn will likely engage the left anterior descending artery.

Anomalous Origin in the Proper Sinus. Another type of anomaly, often involving the right coronary artery, consists of an aberrant origin of the artery within the proper sinus but from an ectopic location. The artery may originate high or low in the sinus, or may originate more posteriorly or anteriorly. Typically, this anomaly is present when the artery is not found in its "usual" location during attempts at selective cannulation with a Judkins catheter. When this form of anomaly affects the right coronary artery, the vessel is often found originating from the aorta at a location higher and more anterior than usual. For the left coronary artery, the vessel often is found in a more posterior position in the sinus. Catheters other than the popular Judkins shape are required to selectively engage these anomalous vessels. The right or left Amplatz catheters are particularly helpful. The only clinical significance of these anomalies relates to their potential for technical difficulties during selective catheter engagement.

Anomalous Origin from a Different Sinus. Anomalous origin of a coronary artery from a different coronary sinus represents a common and important subset of coronary anomalies. In addition to the anomalous origin from the aorta, the proximal segment of the artery often assumes an abnormal course to reach its ultimate destination; importantly, this abnormal path may potentially cause ischemia if it results in acute angulation of the abnormal vessel or if the artery becomes compressed as it winds its way between the aorta and the pulmonary artery. Multiple anomalies have been described and most have no clinical sequelae; however, some specific entities are associated with sudden cardiac death.

Anomalous origin of the left circumflex artery from either the right coronary sinus or directly from the proximal portion of the right coronary artery is one of the most commonly observed coronary anomalies (Figs. 14-3 and 14-4). The anomalous vessel always courses posterior and behind the aorta to reach its ultimate destination. This anomaly is not associated with ischemia or any adverse clinical consequence. The right anterior oblique projection demonstrates the posteriorly directed course of the proximal portion of the artery (Video 14-3). This anomaly should be suspected when selective angiography of the left coronary artery shows the characteristic "long" left main stem with absence of a vessel in the atrioventricular groove (Video 14-4). Although the anomaly may be apparent when selective angiography of the right coronary artery is performed, this is not always the case, particularly if the anomalous vessel originates from the right coronary sinus at some distance from the right coronary artery (Videos 14-5 and 14-6). Usually, the anomalous vessel can be easily engaged with a right Judkins catheter; if this is not successful, a right Amplatz usually succeeds.

The right coronary artery may originate anomalously from the left sinus of Valsalva (Figs. 14-5 and 14-6). This anomaly should be suspected when the right coronary cannot be cannulated at its usual site, there are no collaterals from the left coronary artery, and contrast injection into the right aortic sinus fails to visualize the vessel. A nonselective injection into the left coronary sinus may reveal the right coronary artery (Video 14-7). Most anomalous right coronary arteries from the left coronary sinus course between the aorta and the pulmonary artery. Although somewhat controversial, this anomaly has been associated with myocardial ischemia and sudden cardiac death. These events have been attributed to several mechanisms including acute angulation from its origin, a "slitlike" orifice (see Fig. 14-6), and possibly compression of the vessel by the great vessels during exercise. Selective engagement of these vessels may be difficult; a left Amplatz curve or a short, C-shaped guide catheter may prove successful (Videos 14-8 and 14-9).

Anomalous origin of the left main coronary artery from the right sinus of Valsalva is rare, accounting for roughly 1% of all coronary anomalies detected by angiography. For this anomaly, the left main artery may take one of four possible routes from the right sinus to its ultimate distribution: It may pass *posterior* to the aorta (Fig. 14-7), course *between* the aorta and the pulmonary artery (Fig. 14-8), pass *anterior* to the pulmonary outflow tract (Fig. 14-9), or take an *intraseptal* course to reach its final territory (Fig. 14-10). Of these four variations, anomalous origin of the left main from the right sinus coursing between the aorta and the pulmonary artery is a potentially serious anomaly, and is associated with sudden cardiac death during exertion in young athletes, possibly caused by compression of the artery resulting in ischemia. The other variations are generally believed to be innocent. In one autopsy series (3), the left main passed between the aorta and the pulmonary trunk in the majority of cases (53%) with the posterior course being the next most common variation (23%).

Deciding which variation is present by coronary angiography may be difficult. The right anterior oblique and the 90-degree left lateral projections are helpful in this determination. When the left main courses posteriorly, a distinct, posterior loop is seen in the right anterior oblique projection (Videos 14-10 and 14-11), and the anomalous vessel clearly passes posterior to the catheter in the lateral projection (Fig. 14-11 and Video 14-12). When the left main courses anteriorly, the anomalous vessel makes a clear anterior loop in the right anterior oblique and lateral projections to reach around the pulmonary artery to reach its vascular territory (Videos 14-13 and 14-14; Fig. 14-12). On a left ventriculogram in the straight right anterior oblique projection, an anomalous left main from the right sinus coursing between the aorta and the pulmonary artery often results in the appearance of an anterior "dot" because of the fact that the left main arterial segment is seen "on end" in this view. Selective angiography of this anomaly reveals the absence of either a posterior or anterior loop in the right anterior oblique or lateral views (Video 14-15 and 14-16; Fig. 14-13). Other imaging modalities such as computed tomography and magnetic resonance imaging are helpful to clearly define the course of the anomalous vessel relative to the great arteries.

Variations on this theme occur. A single coronary artery from the right sinus of Valsalva may be present when the entire coronary circulation arises from the right coronary artery (Videos 14-17 and 14-18). Another variation occurs when the individual left coronary arteries (i.e., the left anterior descending and the left circumflex artery) each arise separately from a different location in the right sinus of Valsalva (Videos 14-19 through 14-22).

Anomalous Origin from a Location Other Than the Coronary Sinus. Rarely, the coronary arteries may originate from a location other than the coronary sinus including the pulmonary artery, descending aorta, ascending aorta, or branches of the aorta such as the carotid, innominate artery, or subclavian artery.

Anomalous origin of a coronary artery from the pulmonary artery represents the most significant of these anomalies with major clinical sequelae. The most common of these is anomalous origin of the left coronary from the pulmonary artery (ALCAPA) (Fig. 14-14). This is a serious anomaly. Ninety percent of patients die in infancy, with few surviving to adulthood. The presence of this anomaly in an adult implies a lush collateral network. Angiography reveals an enormous right coronary artery supplying collateral blood to the left coronary artery with reflux of contrast observed into the pulmonary artery (Videos 14-23 and 14-24). In the presence of rich collaterals, ventricular function may be entirely intact. However, this anomaly is associated with sudden cardiac death, myocardial ischemia, and cardiomyopathy, and warrants surgical treatment when discovered. Anomalous origin of the right coronary artery from the pulmonary artery is exceedingly rare (Fig. 14-15). In this anomaly, the left coronary artery supplies collaterals to the right coronary. Angiography of the left coronary artery demonstrates filling of the right coronary artery with reflux of contrast into the pulmonary artery (Videos 14-25 and 14-26).

Other anomalies of this type are relatively benign. An example of an anomalous left coronary artery originating from the ascending aorta is shown in Video 14-27.

Anomalies of Intrinsic Coronary Anatomy

Intrinsic abnormalities of the coronary arterial anatomy compose the second major type of coronary anomalies. These include congenital ectasia or aneurysmal dilation of the artery, absence or hypoplasia of an artery, intramyocardial segments (myocardial "bridge"), and anomalous distributions. The latter two types of anomalies are the most common in this category.

The term *myocardial bridge* is used to describe the presence of an intramyocardial segment of the coronary artery with compression occurring during systole. The true incidence of a myocardial bridge in unselected patients is unclear because they may go unreported unless they are prominent. When present, almost all involve the left anterior descending artery primarily because this vessel lies over a muscular part of the heart (the interventricular septum), whereas the circumflex and right coronaries overlay the coronary sinus in the atrioventricular groove (Video 14-28). Rarely, a bridge may be observed in other arteries (Video 14-29). Myocardial bridges have been associated with myocardial ischemia and sudden cardiac death, but their true significance is not known.

Numerous variations of arterial anatomy caused by anomalous distributions of vessels and their major branches are possible. These anomalies are likely underreported in series of coronary anomalies and, in general, represent benign curiosities. Their major clinical significance lies in the fact that peculiar wall motion abnormalities or unusual electrocardiographic findings may arise when these vessels are involved in an acute myocardial infarction. For instance, the posterior descending artery may originate from the left anterior descending artery "wrapping around" the apex and supplying the entire inferior wall (Fig. 14-16). Thus, acute occlusion of the left anterior descending artery may, in addition to anterior ST-segment elevation, also create inferior ST-segment elevation on an electrocardiogram. This same anomaly can also cause wall motion abnormalities in the inferior wall, as well as the anterior segments with an infarction. These findings would be difficult to reconcile without knowledge of the unique anatomy. The opposite anomaly, where the right coronary artery supplies the apex of the heart from a large posterior descending artery also occurs (see Video 14-19), and acute occlusion of the right coronary artery results in an apical infarction in addition to an inferior event. Ectopic origin of the first septal perforator from the right coronary artery may result in a septal infarction pattern on electrocardiogram in the event of a right coronary occlusion (Video 14-30).

Individual coronary arteries are subject to numerous variations. For example, the circumflex may be absent and instead represent a continuation within the atrioventricular groove of the distal right coronary artery (Fig. 14-17). Similarly, the right coronary artery may be absent or consist solely of a small conus branch with the right coronary artery essentially forming a continuation of the distal circumflex in the atrioventricular groove (Video 14-31).

Another commonly observed anomaly in distribution includes the "split" right coronary artery, where there may either be separate ostia from the aorta for the posterolateral and posterior descending branches, or there is a single ostium but the artery branches very high in the atrioventricular groove (Fig. 14-18; Video 14-32). Numerous variations in anatomy of the left anterior descending artery have been described. There may be a "co-LAD" with two parallel vessels running in the atrioventricular septum with one or both supplying septal perforators, the more lateral branch supplying diagonal arteries, and both supplying the apex. In Video 14-33, a large ramus branch is the dominant vessel supplying the apex and the true "LAD" is a small vessel primarily supplying septal perforators.

Anomalies of Coronary Termination

Abnormalities in coronary artery termination constitute the third major category of coronary anomalies. These primarily consist of fistulous connections between the coronary artery and a cardiac chamber or vascular structure. They are usually small and of little clinical significance. Rarely, they may be large and result in significant shunts or high-output heart failure.

Small, fistulous connections may occur between a coronary artery and any cardiac chamber or structure. The most commonly observed fistula is between the left anterior descending artery and the pulmonary artery (Video 14-34). These are usually small (Video 14-35), without a significant left-to-right shunt, and have little or no clinical consequence. The risk for endocarditis from a small fistula is small. Coronary to pulmonary artery fistulae may also arise from the right coronary artery (Video 14-36) or the left circumflex (Fig. 14-19). Large fistula may result in high-output failure, significant shunting, and progress to aneurysmal dilatation (Video 14-37).

Fistulae can also occur between the coronary artery and one of the cardiac chambers ("coronary cameral" fistula). Not uncommonly, an apparent fistulous connection between the left coronary artery and left ventricle may be observed and often represents a Thebesian network where venous blood from the left coronary distribution drains directly into the left ventricle (video 14-38). These are usually of no clinical consequence, and are associated with hypertensive heart disease and left ventricular hypertrophy. Large coronary cameral fistulae have been associated with myocardial ischemia presumably from a "steal" phenomenon. Intercoronary communications are little more than curiosities. These are sometimes misinterpreted as collateral vessels.

References

1. Yamanaka O, Hobbs RE: Coronary artery anomalies in 126,595 patients undergoing coronary arteriography. Cath Cardiovasc Diagn 1990;21:28–40.
2. Angelini P, Velasco JA, Flamm S: Coronary anomalies: Incidence, pathophysiology, and clinical relevance. Circulation 2002;105:2449–2454.
3. Roberts WC, Shirani J: The four subtypes of anomalous origin of the left coronary artery from the right aortic sinus (or from the right coronary artery). Am J Cardiol 1992;70:119–121.

Normal Origin and Course of Coronary Arteries

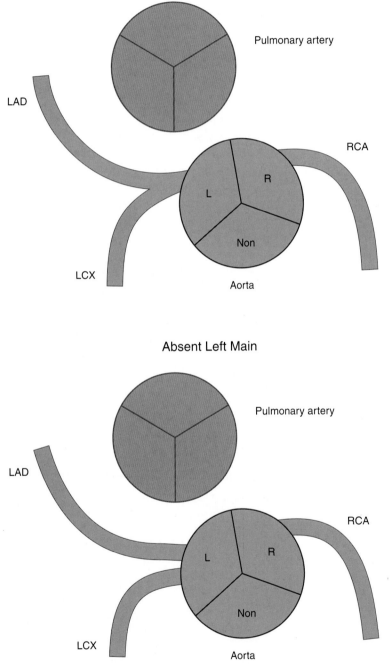

FIGURE 14-1. This cross-sectional view will be used in all subsequent diagrams, and depicts the normal origin and proximal course of the coronary arteries relative to the aorta and pulmonary artery. The direction of view is toward the patient's feet with the ventral surface of the patient at the top. L, left coronary sinus; LAD, left anterior descending artery; LCX, left circumflex; Non, noncoronary cusp; R, right coronary sinus; RCA, right coronary artery.

Absent Left Main

FIGURE 14-2. Absence of the left main. The left circumflex (LCX) and left anterior descending artery (LAD) each arise separately from the left coronary sinus (L). Non, noncoronary cusp; R, right coronary sinus; RCA, right coronary artery.

Anomalous Origin of the LCX from Right Cusp

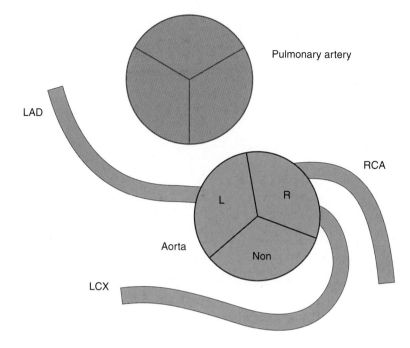

FIGURE 14-3. Depiction of the commonly seen anomalous origin of the left circumflex (LCX) from the right coronary sinus (R). The anomalous vessel passes posteriorly to reach its ultimate vascular territory. L, left coronary sinus; LAD, left anterior descending artery; Non, noncoronary cusp; RCA, right coronary artery.

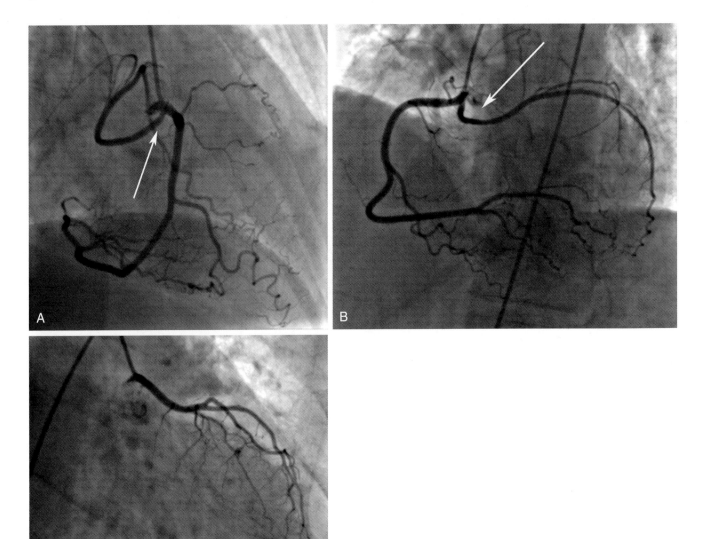

FIGURE 14-4.   Anomalous left circumflex from the right coronary sinus. The right anterior oblique projection *(A)* and left anterior oblique projection *(B)* demonstrate that, in this case, the anomalous left circumflex *(arrow)* arises directly from the proximal segment of the right coronary artery. The left coronary angiogram demonstrates the characteristic appearance of a long left main stem with no vessel within the atrioventricular groove *(C)*.

Anomalous RCA from Left Cusp

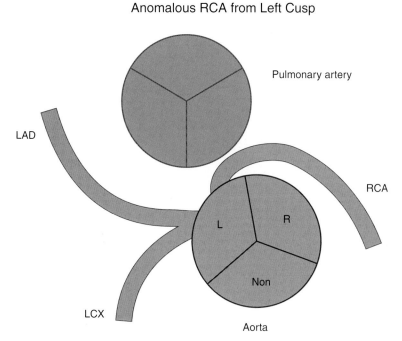

FIGURE 14-5. Depiction of an anomalous origin of the right coronary artery (RCA) from the left (L) or anterior coronary sinus. The anomalous vessel often passes between the pulmonary artery and the aorta to reach its ultimate vascular territory. LAD, left anterior descending artery; LCX, left circumflex; Non, noncoronary cusp; R, right coronary sinus.

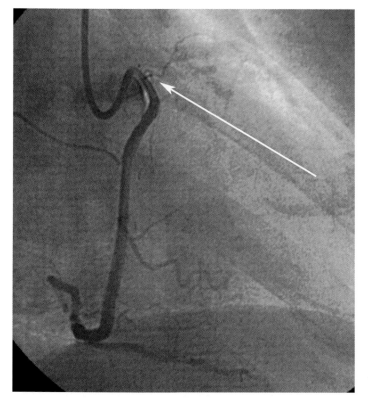

FIGURE 14-6. Anomalous right coronary artery from the left coronary sinus. Notice the "slitlike" orifice (*arrow*) because of the extreme angulation of the proximal segment, and possibly compression between the aorta and the pulmonary artery.

Anomalous Origin of LCA from Right Cusp: Posterior Course

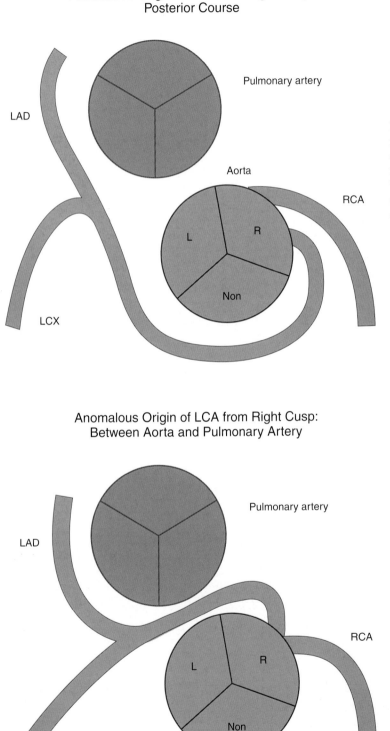

FIGURE 14-7. Anomalous origin of the left coronary artery from the right coronary sinus (R). In this case, the anomalous vessel passes posteriorly to reach its ultimate vascular territory. This variation is benign. L, left coronary sinus; LAD, left anterior descending artery; LCX, left circumflex; Non, noncoronary cusp; RCA, right coronary artery.

Anomalous Origin of LCA from Right Cusp: Between Aorta and Pulmonary Artery

FIGURE 14-8. Anomalous origin of the left coronary artery from the right coronary sinus (R). This variation is potentially life-threatening because the anomalous vessel passes between the pulmonary artery and the aorta to reach its ultimate vascular territory. L, left coronary sinus; LAD, left anterior descending artery; LCX, left circumflex; Non, noncoronary cusp; RCA, right coronary artery.

Anomalous Origin of LCA from Right Cusp: Anterior Course

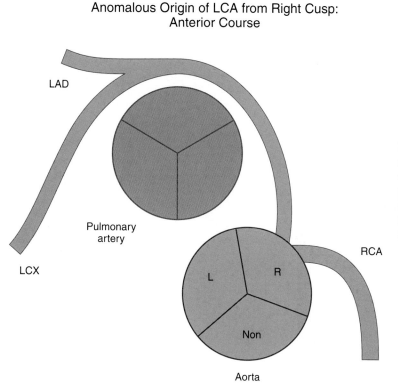

FIGURE 14-9. Anomalous origin of the left coronary artery from the right coronary sinus (R). In this variation, the anomalous vessel passes in front of the pulmonary artery to reach its ultimate vascular territory. L, left coronary sinus; LAD, left anterior descending artery; LCX, left circumflex; Non, noncoronary cusp; RCA, right coronary artery.

Anomalous Origin of LCA from Right Cusp: Septal Course

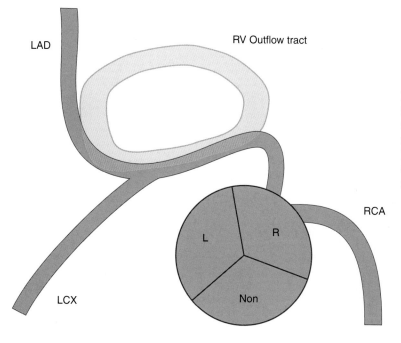

FIGURE 14-10. Anomalous origin of the left coronary artery from the right coronary sinus (R). The anomalous vessel takes a septal course to reach its ultimate vascular territory. L, left coronary sinus; LAD, left anterior descending artery; LCX, left circumflex; Non, noncoronary cusp; RCA, right coronary artery; RV, right ventricular.

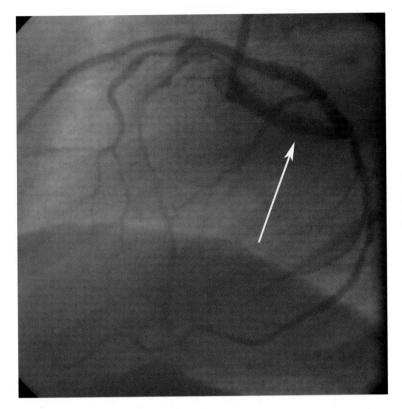

FIGURE 14-11. This angiogram is a left lateral projection demonstrating an anomalous origin of the left main coronary artery (*arrow*) from the right coronary sinus with a posterior course.

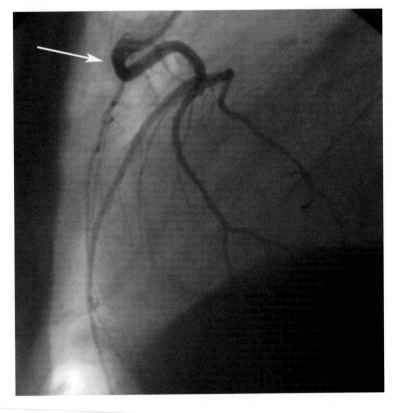

FIGURE 14-12. Left lateral angiogram demonstrating an anomalous origin of the left main coronary artery from the right coronary sinus with an anterior course. Notice the prominent loop (*arrow*) as the anomalous vessel passes in front of the pulmonary artery.

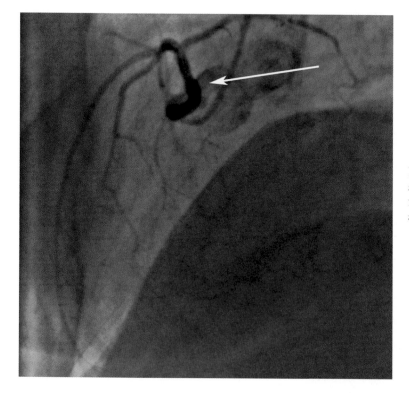

FIGURE 14-13. This left lateral angiogram shows an anomalous left main from the right coronary sinus. The anomalous vessel passes between the aorta and the pulmonary artery.

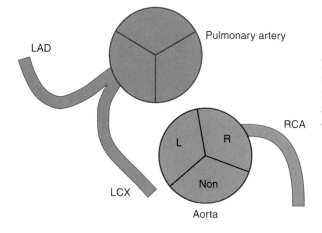

Anomalous Origin of the Left Coronary from the Pulmonary Artery

FIGURE 14-14. Anomalous origin of the left coronary artery from the pulmonary artery. This is a serious anomaly associated with heart failure and sudden cardiac death. L, left coronary sinus; LAD, left anterior descending artery; LCX, left circumflex; Non, noncoronary cusp; R, right coronary sinus; RCA, right coronary artery.

Anomalous Origin and the Right Coronary
from the Pulmonary Artery

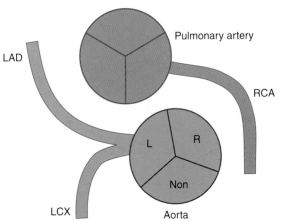

FIGURE 14-15.   This is a depiction of the rarely observed anomalous origin of the right coronary artery (RCA) from the pulmonary artery. L, left coronary sinus; LAD, left anterior descending artery; LCX, left circumflex; Non, noncoronary cusp; R, right coronary sinus.

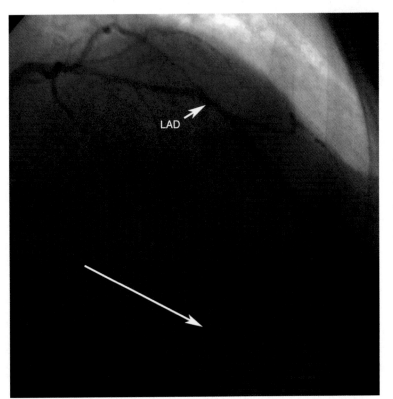

FIGURE 14-16.   Example of a "wrap-around" left anterior descending artery (*LAD*). The apical portion of the LAD is a large vessel supplying the inferior wall and the territory of the posterior descending artery (*arrow*). This patient's right coronary artery primarily supplied a posterolateral branch.

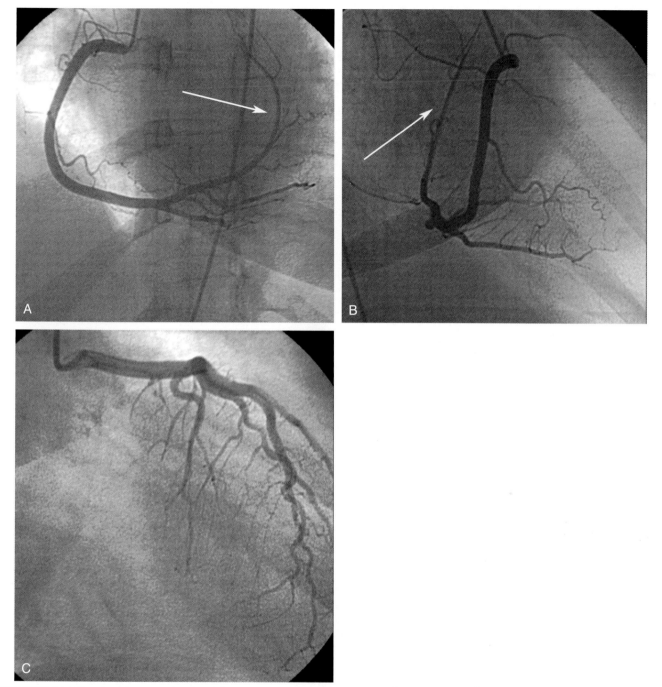

FIGURE 14-17.   In this example, the right coronary artery continues in the atrioventricular groove supplying the circumflex artery as shown in the left anterior oblique view (*A*) and right anterior oblique view (*B*) by the *arrow*. There is no circumflex from the left coronary artery (*C*).

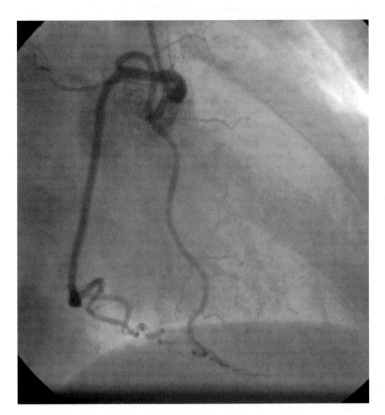

FIGURE 14-18. Example of a split right coronary artery (right anterior oblique view).

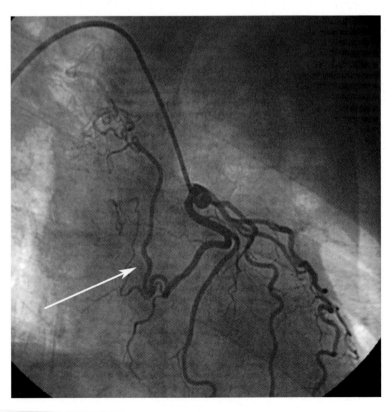

FIGURE 14-19. Most coronary artery to pulmonary artery fistulae arise from the left anterior descending artery or the right coronary artery. In this case, a large fistula originated from the left circumflex.

15

SUPPORT DEVICES

Several important procedures performed in the cardiac catheterization laboratory are used to support a failing heart. The intra-aortic balloon pump (IABP) is an established method of support familiar to all cardiac catheterization laboratories. More recently, greater levels of support became achievable with percutaneous left ventricular assist devices.

Intra-aortic Balloon Pump. The IABP has been used to provide partial circulatory support since its inception in the early 1960s (1,2). The large-profile, early generation devices requiring surgical insertion have been supplanted by the low profile, percutaneous devices currently in use.

The IABP is based on a simple concept. The device consists of a catheter with a long balloon inflating with helium gas to a volume of 30 to 50 mL. The balloon is positioned in the descending aorta and attached to a computerized console regulating the device to inflate during diastole and deflate during systole. This leads to two important beneficial effects on the failing heart: balloon inflation displaces 30 to 50 mL blood augmenting perfusion and increasing diastolic pressure within the aorta (diastolic augmentation), whereas rapid balloon deflation occurring at end-diastole creates a potential space in the aorta, reducing aortic impedance and affording afterload reduction, thereby reducing the work of a failing heart.

The IABP provides only a modest amount of circulatory support. Because the IABP works predominantly by augmenting diastolic pressure and reducing afterload, the device requires some degree of cardiac function to work. Furthermore, optimal timing of inflation and deflation necessitates a stable underlying cardiac rhythm. Therefore, the IABP will not provide effective support in patients with cardiac standstill, tachyarrhythmias, or profoundly reduced systolic function. Importantly, the device is ineffective in noncardiogenic, vasodilatory causes of shock because the 30 to 50 mL blood volume displaced during balloon inflation is simply absorbed by the associated low peripheral vascular resistance preventing pressure augmentation.

Indications for IABP support are listed in Table 15-1. The device is primarily used as a temporary measure of support in patients with cardiogenic shock. It is also frequently used to stabilize patients with severe ischemia and significant coronary artery disease who are awaiting revascularization. Absolute and relative contraindications to an IABP include the presence of severe aortic insufficiency, aortic dissection, aortic aneurysm, severe peripheral vascular disease, marked iliac tortuosity, coagulopathy, and sepsis.

Technique for Insertion and Removal of Intra-aortic Balloon Pump. Percutaneous insertion is easily accomplished from the femoral artery. The IABP catheter arrives prepackaged from the manufacturer with all necessary equipment, requiring minimal preparation before use. Just before insertion, the catheter is removed from the package, placed on a sterile field, and the central lumen flushed. A one-way valve is attached to the balloon port and aspirated with a syringe to maintain the balloon under negative pressure. Using sterile technique, the operator administers local anesthesia and punctures the common femoral artery with an arterial access needle. Most IABP kits include the appropriate guide wires and sheaths compatible with the

Table 15-1.	Selected Indications for Intra-aortic Balloon Pump Support

Postmyocardial infarction shock
  Severe pump failure
  Mechanic complication (papillary muscle rupture, acute ventricular septal defect)

Decompensated heart failure

Severe, acute mitral regurgitation

Unstable angina refractory to medical therapy or before coronary bypass surgery in high-risk patients

Decompensated aortic stenosis

Refractory ventricular tachycardia

Support of high-risk percutaneous coronary intervention (PCI)

Threatened closure from PCI requiring emergency bypass surgery

balloon catheter. It is worth noting that the central lumen of the balloon pump catheter requires a 0.030- or 0.032-inch J-tipped guide wire and not the standard-sized 0.035-inch guide wire used routinely for cardiac catheterizations. It is helpful to observe the course of the guide wire through the iliac arteries under fluoroscopy; severe iliac tortuosity may preclude advancement of an IABP catheter (Fig. 15-1). If severe peripheral vascular disease is suspected, an abdominal aortogram should first be performed to determine the suitability of the iliac and femoral vessels for this procedure. Once the guide wire is situated in the descending aorta, an appropriately sized sheath (current designs allow an 8 French sheath) is inserted and the sheath's dilator removed, leaving the guide wire in place. Under fluoroscopic guidance, the balloon pump catheter is advanced over the guide wire until the radio-opaque marker reaches the level of the left mainstem bronchus (Fig. 15-2). The guide wire is removed and blood aspirated from the catheter lumen, then flushed with heparinized saline and connected to the console's pressure transducer. The balloon port is connected by tubing to the console and the balloon filled with helium gas. Observing inflation and deflation of the balloon under fluoroscopy ensures that the balloon is unwrapping fully without kinks or obstructions to filling. Systemic heparin is often administered to prevent thrombus formation on the balloon and catheter.

The effectiveness of the IABP depends on proper timing of inflation and deflation. For optimal performance, the balloon is timed to rapidly inflate just after the dicrotic notch, indicating aortic valve closure and is set to rapidly deflate just before aortic ejection. Adjustments to timing are usually made with counterpulsation set at 2:1 (i.e., two complete cardiac cycles for every one balloon inflation/deflation cycle). Figure 15-3 presents an example of optimal timing. The pressure increase with balloon inflation beginning at the dicrotic notch creates an increase in diastolic pressure known as the *augmentation wave*. Ideal timing for deflation is noted as an end-diastolic pressure of the augmented waveform lower than the end-diastolic pressure of a nonaugmented beat.

Incorrect timing causes, at minimum, inefficient counterpulsation but may even lead to deleterious effects on cardiac function. If the balloon is inflated when the aortic valve is still open (early inflation), the associated increase in pressure causes early closure of the aortic valve impairing ventricular emptying and decreasing stroke volume. Aortic regurgitation may also occur, increasing the work of the heart. Late deflation is also detrimental because ventricular ejection begins against an increased aortic impedence having unfavorable effects on myocardial oxygen demand, stroke volume, and cardiac output. Arrhythmias, particularly atrial fibrillation, multifocal atrial tachycardia, and frequent ventricular ectopy, interfere with proper timing of the IABP and are a cause of ineffective counterpulsation.

Post-Intra-aortic Balloon Pump Patient Care. Once an IABP is inserted, the patient is placed in an intensive care unit on strict bed rest unable to flex the hip joint more than 20 degrees. Frequent examination of the catheter insertion site, distal pulses, and lower extremity perfusion is important for prevention of serious vascular complications. Most clinicians maintain patients with an IABP on therapeutic levels of intravenous heparin unless contraindicated.

In most cases, if an IABP is inserted before surgery or percutaneous revascularization, the device can be quickly removed once this goal is accomplished. Patients with cardiogenic shock or severe heart failure require gradual weaning of support. This can begin as soon as a patient has demonstrated hemodynamic stability evidenced by adequate blood pressure and cardiac output, and no significant pulmonary congestion. The process can be facilitated by using inotropic or vasopressor support in patients with tenuous hemodynamics. Weaning is initiated by decreasing counterpulsation from 1:1 to 1:2. After 2 to 4 hours, if there is no evidence of decompensation and continued hemodynamic stability, support can be decreased to 1:4. Removal of the IABP can occur if there is continued clinical stability after a period of observation on 1:4 counterpulsation.

To remove an IABP, the operator discontinues anticoagulation and places the pump on a 1:4 or 1:8 counterpulsation ratio to prevent clot formation. After administration of local anesthetic, the catheter is disconnected from the console and suction is applied with a syringe to collapse the balloon. Once inflated, the IABP balloon retains a high profile and cannot be withdrawn through the sheath. Removal requires that the balloon catheter and sheath are removed together as one unit. Because small clots may form on the balloon catheter and potentially occlude the femoral artery, the puncture site is allowed to bleed freely for a second or two to help expel any thrombus inadvertently dragged into the access site. Hemostasis is achieved by manual compression of the arteriotomy site for 30 to 60 minutes, and a sterile dressing is applied. The patient should remain at bed rest for several hours to prevent rebleeding.

Complications of Intra-aortic Balloon Pump. Earlier generations experienced high complication rates with percutaneous insertion of the IABP. Recent advances in technology and adoption of smaller caliber catheters have greatly improved the safety profile of this apparatus. Nevertheless, there remains potential for major complications from this important device (Table 15-2) (3).

Table 15-2.	Complications of Intra-aortic Balloon Pump

Vascular Complications

Access site bleeding

Hematoma

Retroperitoneal bleeding

Vessel injury/perforation

Aortic dissection

Pseudoaneurysm

Arterial insufficiency
   Asymptomatic loss of pulses
   Acute limb ischemia

Infection

Local wound infection

Bacteremia/sepsis

Rare Complications

Lymphedema

Femoral cutaneous nerve damage

Cerebrovascular accident

Hemolysis

Thrombocytopenia

Helium embolism

Vascular entrapment of balloon

Spinal cord necrosis and paraplegia

Mesenteric/renal/splenic infarction

The most commonly observed complications are vascular in nature and include bleeding, hematoma, arterial injury, pseudoaneurysm, and acute limb ischemia. Acute limb ischemia is a serious and potentially limb-threatening complication. A spectrum exists from asymptomatic loss of the distal arterial pulses to profound ischemia and tissue loss. Symptoms of acute ischemia include limb pain, paresthesias, or loss of motor or sensory function with the physical examination revealing diminished or absent pulses, pallor, and coolness of the extremity. The mechanism of IABP-induced limb ischemia is most commonly due to mechanical obstruction of the arterial lumen from the large-bore sheath and catheter in the presence of small arteries or preexisting peripheral vascular disease. Other explanations include thrombus, embolism, or arterial dissection created during device insertion. If removal of the balloon pump does not promptly restore circulation to the threatened limb, urgent vascular surgery consultation is needed because a surgical procedure may be required.

Other complications listed in Table 15-2 are uncommon. A rare, but noteworthy complication occurs when small leaks or tears arise in the balloon and blood is observed in the helium tube connecting the catheter to the console. When this occurs, the balloon must be promptly removed because the blood may desiccate and prevent the balloon from deflating, entrapping the catheter and making it impossible to remove percutaneously.

Percutaneous Left Ventricular Assist Devices. Percutaneous left ventricular assist devices are relatively recent additions to the armamentarium of the cardiac catheterization laboratory designed to overcome many of the important limitations of the IABP. These devices offer levels of circulatory support not achievable with an IABP.

The TandemHeart (CardiacAssist, Pittsburg, PA) is currently the most widely used percutaneous left ventricular assist device providing flow rates of up to 5 L/min. Oxygenated blood is pumped from the left atrium to the arterial circulation in a nonpulsatile, continuous manner using a small, extracorporeal centrifugal pump (Fig. 15-4). The 21 Fr left atrial catheter is placed percutaneously using a trans-septal approach from the right femoral vein. Blood is returned through a 15 to 17 French arterial catheter placed percutaneously into the common femoral artery, and patients are maintained on high levels of systemic anticoagulation to prevent thrombus formation.

The TandemHeart is most commonly used to support high-risk, percutaneous cardiac procedures. This form of support is ideal for patients with severely reduced left ventricular function about to undergo a complex percutaneous coronary intervention on the left main coronary artery or other major artery supplying a large vascular territory. In such instances, ischemia occurring during the intervention may lead to devastating consequences including cardiovascular collapse, refractory arrhythmias, and death. Circulatory support is needed only for the duration of the procedure, allowing the operator to proceed with confidence that vital organ perfusion will be maintained in the event of transient cardiovascular collapse during the intervention. Examples of other procedures supported by percutaneous left ventricular assist devices include aortic balloon valvuloplasty, percutaneous aortic valve replacement, ablation of ventricular tachycardia, high-risk rotational atherectomy, and bypass surgery.

The other main indication is for support of a failing heart. The device has been shown to increase cardiac output, increase mean arterial pressure, and reduce pulmonary capillary wedge pressure in patients in cardiogenic shock or refractory heart failure (4). It is particularly useful to correct life- or organ-threatening hemodynamic abnormalities in patients with reversible causes of shock or heart failure such as acute myocardial infarction, myocarditis, or cardiac transplant rejection. It serves as a method to "bridge" a critically ill patient to cardiac transplant or a more durable, surgical left ventricular assist device.

In most patients, full circulatory support is available within an hour of beginning the procedure. Venous access is obtained initially with a 7 Fr sheath from the right femoral vein and a right-heart catheterization performed to assess baseline filling pressures and cardiac output. Low left atrial pressure prevents adequate pump function; therefore, if filling pressures are low, fluid boluses should be administered. Arterial access is generally obtained from the left femoral artery; initially, a 6 Fr sheath is placed. Angiography of the distal aorta and iliacs is often performed to assess the size of the iliac and femoral vessels, and determine the presence of peripheral vascular disease that might preclude use of the device. When the operator is satisfied, the console, pump, and cannulae may be prepared for use and set aside in the sterile field.

The trans-septal cannulation is performed first. A routine trans-septal puncture is performed, and a stiff but floppy-tipped 0.035-inch guide wire is placed in the left atrium. The skin tract and atrial septum are dilated with a two-stage dilator over the guide wire. The dilator is removed and a 14 Fr obturator inserted into the 21 Fr cannula, and advanced over the wire and across the atrial septum. The 21 Fr trans-septal cannula has 14 holes at the distal end, and these should all be within the left atrium and position confirmed by fluoroscopy (Fig. 15-5). When the cannula is satisfactorily positioned, the guide wire and obturator may be removed and the proximal end of the tubing clamped. The cannula is labeled with numbers marking the depth in centimeters of insertion. The depth marking at the skin level should be noted by the operator serving as a monitor for cannula movement.

With the trans-septal cannula in place, systemic heparin is administered to achieve activated clotting time longer than 400 seconds. The 6 Fr arterial sheath is then replaced with a 15 or 17 Fr arterial cannula depending on the size of the iliac and femoral vessels over an 0.035-inch guide wire and after first dilating the tissue tract with smaller caliber dilators. The proximal end of the arterial cannula is clamped. The centrifugal pump is primed and placed on the patient's right thigh, and the trans-septal and arterial cannulae connected. Once all air bubbles have been removed from the system, the clamps may be released and circulatory support initiated.

While the pump is in use, it is important to maintain adequate levels of anticoagulation with systemic heparinization to prevent thrombus formation. The patient is placed on strict bed rest and moved only with the greatest of care to prevent cannula dislodgement. Sedation forms an important component of patient management during use of the device. Flow rates are continuously monitored and maintained at the desired level with a maximum achievable flow of about 5 L/min. Flow rates are sensitive to left atrial volume and decreased flows often respond to fluid boluses.

Percutaneous left ventricular assist devices are intended for short-term use. When used to support a high-risk coronary intervention, the device is needed for only a few hours. In patients with cardiogenic shock or refractory heart failure, support may be needed for several days. Once a patient no longer requires support, the device may be removed. The tubing is first clamped and the device turned off. The trans-septal cannula is withdrawn and manual pressure applied to the femoral vein access site until hemostasis achieved. Similarly, the arterial cannula is removed and manual pressure applied. Prolonged compression using commercially available devices may assist in achieving hemostasis and limit bleeding complications. When the device is used only in the cardiac catheterization laboratory to support a procedure, arterial hemostasis may be achieved by deploying a suture-mediated closure device at the time of access; this technique should not be used for prolonged insertions because of the risk for infection. Vascular surgical assistance is sometimes required if difficulty with hemostasis is anticipated.

The device's requirement for large arterial cannulae precludes its use in the presence of severe peripheral vascular disease or small (<5-mm) iliac arteries. Patients with severe right-heart failure are unlikely to benefit if there is poor right-sided cardiac output, and pump performance is suboptimal whenever there is low left atrial pressure. This may occur in the setting of bleeding, hypovolemia, cardiac arrest, and pulmonary hypertension. Patients with sustained and rapid atrial or ventricular arrhythmia may experience diminished flow rates from impaired right-heart output. Other potential contraindications include severe aortic insufficiency and inability to anticoagulate because of bleeding.

Complications of the device include access-site bleeding, arterial injury during cannula insertion, acute limb ischemia, and complications related to trans-septal puncture. Air embolism may occur when connecting the device to the trans-septal cannula if left atrial pressure is low. Dislodgement of the trans-septal cannula is a serious complication often occurring if the patient moves, is carelessly transported, or receives cardiopulmonary resuscitation. This problem is identified by a rapid decline in oxygen saturation and the discovery of dark blood instead of bright red blood in the pump tubing. This problem requires the physician to reposition the cannula in the left atrium or device removal.

References

1. Moulopoulos SD, Topaz S, Kolff WJ: Diastolic balloon pumping (with carbon dioxide) in the aorta: A mechanical assistance to the failing circulation. Am Heart J 1962;63:669–675.
2. Kantrowitz A, Tjonneland S, Freed PS, et al: Initial clinical experience with intra-aortic balloon pumping in cardiogenic shock. JAMA 1968;203:135–140.
3. Trost JC, Hillis LD: Intra-aortic balloon counterpulsation. Am J Cardiol 2006;97:1391–1398.
4. Thiele H, Lauer B, Hambrecht R, et al: Reversal of cardiogenic shock by percutaneous left atrial-to-femoral arterial bypass assistance. Circulation 2001;104:2917–2922.

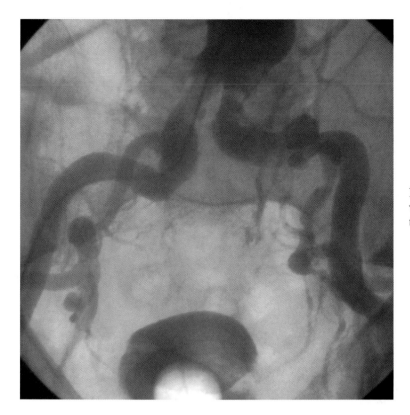

FIGURE 15-1. Severe, bilateral iliac tortuosity prevented insertion of an intra-aortic balloon pump in this patient.

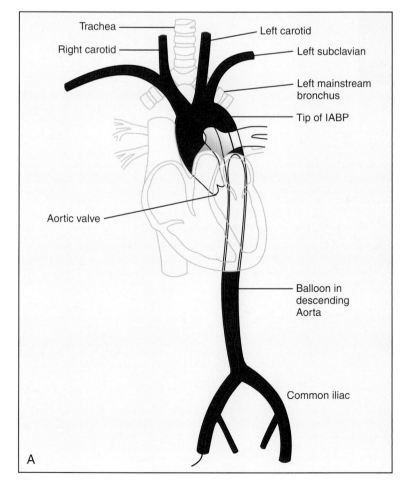

FIGURE 15-2. *A,* Relation between the tip of the balloon pump, the left subclavian artery, and the left mainstem bronchus.

Continued

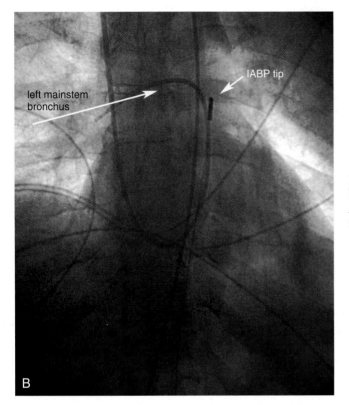

FIGURE 15-2. cont'd   *B*, Radiographic appearance of the balloon pump in the proper location in the descending aorta. *Arrow* shows the location of the left mainstem bronchus. IABP, intra-aortic balloon pump.

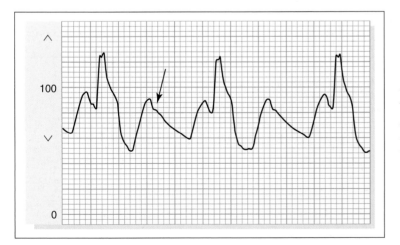

FIGURE 15-3.   Optimal timing of the intra-aortic balloon pump. *Arrow* shows the location of the dicrotic notch. The balloon should inflate just after the dicrotic notch and should be fully deflated before the next ejection begins.

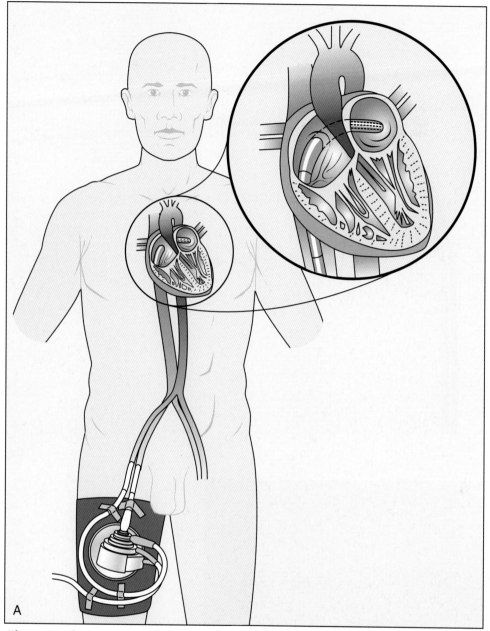

FIGURE 15-4. The essential components of the TandemHeart (CardiacAssist, Pittsburgh, PA) percutaneous left ventricular assist device are shown. A 21 French (Fr) cannula is placed trans-septally into the left atrium, and a pump draws oxygenated blood from the left atrium to the iliac arteries delivering up to 5 L/min blood flow (A).

Continued

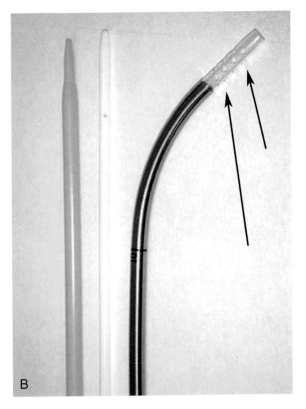

FIGURE 15-4. cont'd *B*, Detail of the trans-septal cannula system. The blue dilator is used first to create a suitable passage. The white dilator is placed within the 21 Fr cannula (far right) and removed when the cannula is in its final position in the left atrium. Note the multiple side holes on the trans-septal cannula *(arrow)*; these should all be well within the left atrium during surgery.

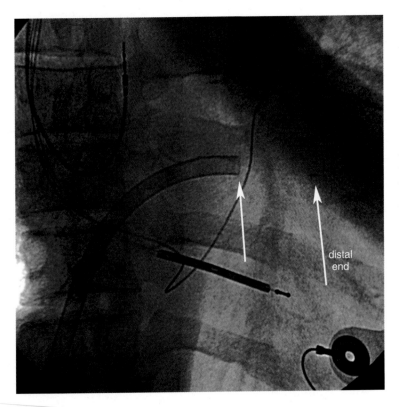

FIGURE 15-5. Fluoroscopic appearance of the 21 French (Fr) cannula properly positioned within the left atrium for use with the TandemHeart (CardiacAssist, Pittsburgh, PA) percutaneous left ventricular assist device. The radiolucent section between the *arrows* contains the inlet holes. This section should remain entirely within the left atrium for proper functioning.

CHAPTER 16

PERICARDIOCENTESIS AND BALLOON PERICARDIAL WINDOW

Pericardial effusions occur commonly from multiple causative agents (Table 16-1). In the United States, viral pericarditis, iatrogenic effusions from coronary or cardiac chamber perforation during an interventional procedure, malignancy, and idiopathic pericarditis are the most common of these causes. Small- or moderate-sized effusions without associated hemodynamic consequences usually require no further therapy. Large or small effusions that cause significant hemodynamic compromise require drainage. Pericardiocentesis is also indicated when diagnosis of the effusion requires analysis of the pericardial fluid.

Pericardiocentesis. Clinically stable patients who require percutaneous drainage of a pericardial effusion ideally undergo pericardiocentesis in the cardiac catheterization laboratory. The procedure may be performed emergently at the bedside in a critically ill patient whose condition is rapidly deteriorating from tamponade and who is unable to be transported to the cardiac catheterization laboratory. In preparation for the procedure, the operator reviews pertinent laboratory values including prothrombin time, partial thromboplastin time, platelet count, and electrolytes. Consent should include a description of the complications of the procedure (described later) and the possibility that the procedure will not successfully drain the effusion.

Before performing pericardiocentesis, it is helpful for the operator to carefully review the echocardiogram (Fig. 16-1). The subcostal view demonstrates the path the needle must take to reach the effusion from the subxiphoid approach and provides an estimate of the distance to the fluid. Furthermore, echocardiography helps the operator identify a route that avoids the liver or other structures and clearly demonstrates the size of the effusion. Small effusions that cause tamponade may be quite challenging to drain percutaneously, particularly in obese individuals. Excessive "stranding" or texturing within the fluid provides an important clue suggesting loculation of the fluid. Based on the echocardiogram, the operator may choose an apical or even parasternal approach as an alternative to the subxiphoid entry.

During the procedure, the rhythm and oxygen saturation are monitored continuously. Advanced cardiac life support and skilled technical and nursing staff should be readily available in the event of an arrhythmia or respiratory arrest. Careful assessment of right-heart pressures before and after pericardiocentesis offers valuable insight. Characteristic hemodynamic abnormalities of tamponade include increased and equalized right chamber diastolic pressures, a low cardiac output, and an initial pericardial pressure equal to right atrial pressure. If these abnormalities are absent, the effusion may not be hemodynamically significant

Table 16-1.	Selected Causes of Pericardial Effusions

Infection

Bacterial
  Streptococcus, Staphylococcus, gram-negative rods

Mycobacterial
  Tuberculosis

Viral
  Coxsackie, echovirus, adenovirus, Ebstein–Barr virus
  Human immunodeficiency virus

Fungal
  Aspergillosis, Candida, histoplasmosis

Protozoal
  Amebic

Neoplastic

Primary mesothelioma

Metastatic
  Breast, lung, skin, lymphoma, leukemia

Metabolic

Uremia, myxedema, amyloidosis

Immune/Inflammatory

Connective tissue disorders (lupus, scleroderma, Polyarteritis nodosa (PAN),
  rheumatoid arthritis)

Sarcoidosis

After myocardial infarction, postpericardiotomy syndrome

Iatrogenic

Radiation induced

Cardiac perforation from interventional procedures

Drugs (warfarin [Coumadin], minoxidil, procainamide)

Trauma

Direct trauma

Aortic dissection

Idiopathic

or fully explain the patient's clinical syndrome. With successful pericardiocentesis, the right-sided pressures return to normal and pericardial pressure declines to zero or less. Demonstration of persistent hemodynamic abnormalities after pericardiocentesis indicates the presence of other heart or lung pathology, loculation of pericardial fluid, or the presence of effusive constrictive pericarditis.

Pericardiocentesis is most commonly performed from the subxiphoid approach. The procedure is facilitated by positioning the patient at 30 to 45 degrees; this allows fluid to collect inferiorly and posteriorly. After preparing the area with sterile technique, the skin around the left side of the xiphoid process at the costal angle is anesthetized with 10 mL of 2% lidocaine. A 4- to 5-mm skin nick is made and the tissue tract dilated with a hemostat. An additional 10 mL of 2% lidocaine is administered more deeply to the level of the pericardium.

The pericardial sac usually lies an average of 4 to 6 cm below the skin from the subxiphoid approach. Thus, entry into the pericardial space usually requires a long (10–12-cm) needle outfitted with a solid stylet to prevent tissue from plugging the needle lumen. These are usually provided in the commercially available pericardiocentesis kits with the other needed equipment. From the left costoxiphoid angle, the needle is advanced at a 30-degree angle and directed toward the left shoulder. Once the needle tip penetrates the subcutaneous tissue and passes below the rib, the angle of the needle is flattened to about 15 to 20 degrees and advanced. Several distinct "pops" are felt as the needle passes through the deep fascia of the chest wall and the parietal pericardium. When the operator believes the needle tip is within the pericardial space, the stylet is removed. Fluid return (especially straw colored) usually indicates successful entry into the pericardial space. At this point, the needle is attached to a pressure transducer, and simultaneous right atrial and pericardial pressure is recorded; these two pressures are usually equal in tamponade (Fig. 16-2). Depending on the cause, pericardial fluid may be bloody; but a bloody return may also indicate inadvertent entry into the right ventricle. For this reason, analysis of the pressure waveform sampled from the needle tip helps confirm the correct location within the pericardial space.

With the needle in the pericardial space, a 0.035-inch J-tipped guidewire is advanced under fluoroscopic guidance. The wire course should lie within the confines of the pericardium (Fig. 16-3) and not along the pulmonary artery or pleural cavity. When it is difficult to establish whether the needle has unequivocally entered the pericardium, demonstration of a contrast effect within the pericardial space on transthoracic echocardiography performed during an injection of agitated saline through the needle confirms the proper location. The needle should be repositioned if contrast appears within the right ventricle.

A 5 or 6 French (Fr) dilator is advanced over the guide wire, removed, and replaced with a pigtail catheter positioned under fluoroscopy. The wire is withdrawn and fluid aspirated. Pericardial pressure is remeasured when fluid can no longer be aspirated. Ideally, a successful pericardiocentesis achieves a pericardial pressure of zero. Clinical signs indicating successful relief of tamponade include a decrease in right atrial pressure, restoration of blood pressure, loss of pulsus paradox, and an increase in cardiac output. If the pericardial pressure does not decrease to zero, a loculated effusion may be present. Effusive constrictive pericarditis is suggested by a decline in pericardial pressure but continued increase of right atrial pressure and prominence of the "y" descent (Fig. 16-4).

In many cases, the cause of the pericardial effusions is clear and no further workup is needed. Patients with effusion of unknown cause undergo evaluation including a careful history and physical examination, chest radiograph, and possibly abdominal and chest computed tomography and routine blood tests for common hematologic, rheumatologic, metabolic, and endocrine abnormalities. Pericardial fluid analysis (cell count, glucose, Gram stain, culture, and cytologic examination) may provide additional insight (1, 2). The yield is greatest for infection or malignancy. Unlike pleural effusions, distinction between a transudate and exudate is not helpful because many cases of pericardial effusion caused by heart failure are exudative. Furthermore, contrary to popular belief, no diagnostic value exists in the presence of a hemorrhagic effusion. Benign causes may be hemorrhagic and malignancies may be straw colored and clear. Note that fluid analysis is rarely diagnostic of mycobacterial infection; these diagnoses usually require pericardial tissue biopsy.

Overall, pericardiocentesis is a safe procedure. Complications include arrhythmia, pneumothorax, injury to liver or adjacent structures, failure to completely relieve tamponade because of loculation, recurrence of effusion, infection, and hemopericardium from chamber perforation or coronary artery laceration.

Depending on the cause of the effusion, the pericardial catheter can be removed once the fluid is completely drained. A pericardial drain may be left in place for up to 24 to 48 hours when concern exists about rapid reaccumulation of fluid. When a drain remains in the pericardial space, careful attention to sterility is important and the catheter requires regular flushing under sterile conditions every 1 to 2 hours using a few milliliters of heparinized saline to prevent occlusion. If there is no significant drainage or reaccumulation of fluid, the catheter should be removed as soon as possible to prevent infection.

In experienced hands, pericardiocentesis can also be performed from the apical approach if the effusion is not accessible from a subxiphoid one. This technique requires echocardiographic guidance to localize the site on the chest where the effusion is in closest contact with the chest wall without intervening lung or rib. Positioning the patient partly on his or her left side in a semirecumbent fashion facilitates access to the effusion. Needle passage should occur over the top of the rib to avoid the neurovascular bundle.

Balloon Pericardial Window. Recurrent effusion is an important limitation to pericardiocentesis. Recurrence is particularly problematic for patients with malignant effusions, in whom life expectancy is limited and great value placed in time free from hospital admissions and medical procedures. Percutaneous balloon pericardiotomy evolved from the desire to offer a less invasive alternative to the traditional surgical pericardial window for palliation of recurrent malignant pericardial effusions (3, 4).

Under local anesthesia, a balloon pericardial window is performed by using a valvuloplasty balloon at the time of pericardiocentesis to create a tear in the pericardium. This allows drainage of pericardial fluid into the pleural or peritoneal space, or both, preventing reaccumulation of pericardial fluid and the associated, potentially deleterious hemodynamic consequences. This procedure is most effective in patients with malignant effusions and should be avoided in patients with uremic pericarditis because of increased risk for bleeding. In a multicenter registry involving 130 patients with mostly malignant pericardial effusion, balloon pericardial window was successful in 85% of patients, defined as no recurrence or need for surgery (1). The procedure was unsuccessful in 18 patients (15%) and consisted of bleeding requiring surgery in 5 patients (all of whom had uremic pericardial effusions) and recurrence in 13 patients.

The procedure should be avoided in patients with active infections in the overlying tissues or pericardial space and in those with significant coagulopathy. Balloon pericardial window may not be effective in individuals with large left pleural effusions preventing adequate drainage to the left pleural space or in those who have had extensive chest radiation or surgical scarring because these conditions may interfere with fluid reabsorption.

The operator begins by first performing a pericardiocentesis using the subxiphoid approach in the manner described. The potential exists for significant procedural pain; thus, it is important to provide liberal sedation and local anesthesia. Once the pericardial space is entered and tamponade relieved, a 0.038-inch "extra-stiff" J-wire is passed into the pericardial space and the pigtail catheter removed. A 10 Fr dilator is passed over the wire to create a suitable skin and tissue tract. A valvuloplasty balloon (3–4 cm long and 20 mm in diameter) is prepared using dilute contrast and passed along the wire into the pericardial space. At this point, the patient should be placed fully recumbent to prevent kinking of the catheter and allow easier passage.

It is important to position the balloon properly across the pericardium to create a suitable tear in the pericardium. The entire balloon should be below the skin and the balloon centered across the inferior pericardial border. Using a 60-mL syringe, the balloon is gently inflated under fluoroscopic guidance. A "waist" should be evident where the balloon crosses the pericardium. With increasing pressure, dilation should continue until the balloon is fully expanded (Fig. 16-5). Once accomplished, the balloon can be removed over the guide wire and replaced with the pigtail catheter to remove any residual fluid.

The catheter is usually removed and an occlusive (air-tight) dressing applied to the wound. After the procedure, a chest roentgenogram is obtained to assess for the presence of pneumothorax or pleural effusion. Complications include all of those noted for pericardiocentesis. In addition, complications unique to percutaneous balloon pericardiotomy include significant pleural effusion, pneumothorax, hemopericardium, hemothorax, infection, and periprocedural pain.

Pericardial Fluoroscopy. During cardiac catheterization, fluoroscopy may reveal pericardial calcification. This finding, together with the characteristic hemodynamic findings, may support a diagnosis of constrictive pericarditis. However, variable degrees of pericardial calcification may also be observed after heart surgery without evidence of pericardial constraint (Video 16-1). The significance of this unusual finding is not clear.

References

1. Wiener HG, Kristensen IB, Haubek A, et al: The diagnostic value of pericardial cytology: An analysis of 95 cases. Acta Cytol 1991;35:149–153.
2. Corey GR, Campbell PT, Van Trigt P, et al: Etiology of large pericardial effusions. Am J Med 1993;95:209–213.
3. Ziskind AA, Lemmon CC, Rodriguez S, et al: Final report of the Percutaneous Balloon Pericardiotomy Registry for the Treatment of Effusive Pericardial Disease. Circulation 1994;90:I-647A.
4. Ziskind AA, Pearce AC, Lemmon CC, et al: Percutaneous balloon pericardiotomy for the treatment of cardiac tamponade and large pericardial effusions: Description of technique and report of the first 50 cases. J Am Coll Cardiol 1993;21:1–5.

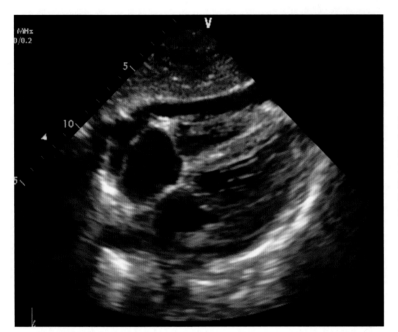

FIGURE 16-1. This transthoracic echocardiogram was obtained from a subcostal acoustic window and demonstrates a circumferential pericardial effusion. Note that a lobe of the liver lies between the skin surface and the effusion. The needle will take a similar path when pericardiocentesis is performed in this patient from a subxiphoid approach.

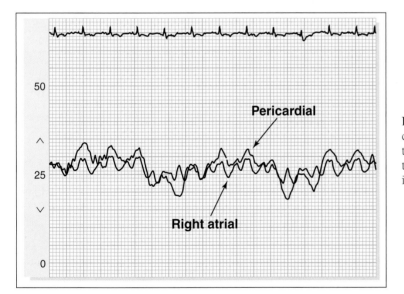

FIGURE 16-2. Simultaneous right atrial and pericardial pressures obtained during right-heart catheterization and pericardiocentesis in a patient with tamponade. Note that there is an increase and equalization of these pressures.

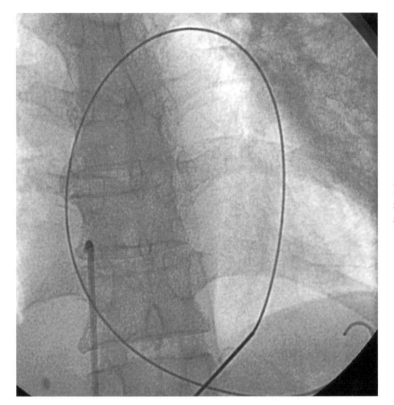

FIGURE 16-3. Once a needle enters the pericardial space, a 0.035-inch J-tipped guide wire is advanced, and its course should take the appearance shown here.

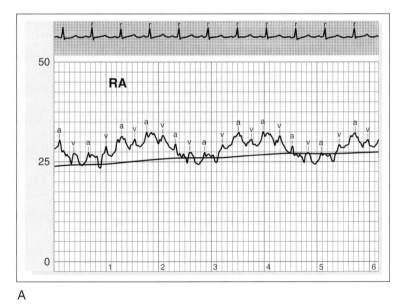

A

FIGURE 16-4. These tracings were obtained in a patient with effusive constrictive pericarditis. Before pericardiocentesis, the right atrial (RA) pressure is increased, and the "x" and "y" descents are attenuated (A).

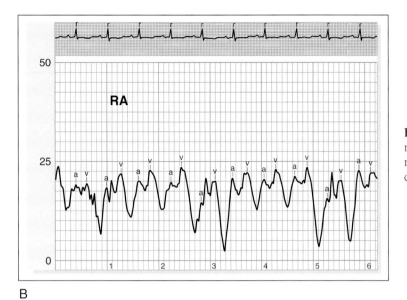

FIGURE 16-4. cont'd   After pericardiocentesis with removal of all pericardial fluid, the right atrial pressure remains increased with prominence of the "x" and "y" descents (*B*).

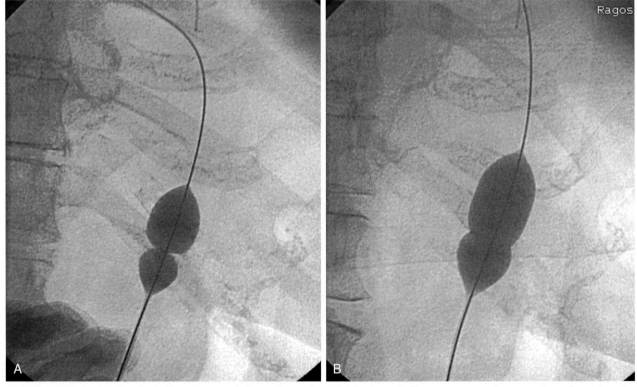

FIGURE 16-5.   Example of a balloon pericardial window. The valvuloplasty balloon is centered across the inferior border of the pericardium (*A*) with a prominent waste present at the site the balloon enters the pericardial space. Full inflation causes a tear in the pericardial sac at the site of the original waist (*B*).

CHAPTER 17

ENDOMYOCARDIAL BIOPSY

Percutaneous biopsy of the myocardium is a well-established technique performed in the cardiac catheterization laboratory. Most of these procedures consist of right ventricular biopsy. Left ventricular biopsy is only rarely performed either to sample tumors within the left ventricle or to define the presence of specific processes confined to the left ventricle.

Right ventricular endomyocardial biopsy is most commonly used to determine the presence of rejection in patients who have undergone cardiac transplantation. A paucity of data exists supporting this procedure for indications outside of this subset. Recently published expert guidelines describe several clinical scenarios (Table 17-1) in which the results from myocardial biopsy may provide important prognostic data or lead to changes in patient management (1). The greatest enthusiasm (Class I and Class IIa recommendations) for this procedure involved patients with unexplained, new-onset heart failure in whom the clinical course is suspicious for specific types of myocarditis (lymphocytic, giant-cell, hypersensitivity, or necrotizing eosinophilic myocarditis), sarcoidosis, anthracycline cardiomyopathy, restrictive cardiomyopathy, or a cardiac tumor. In addition, endomyocardial biopsy may be performed as part of a research protocol.

Technique. Endomyocardial biopsy is performed in the cardiac catheterization laboratory with fluoroscopic guidance by experienced operators. Right-heart catheterization is typically performed before the biopsy. During the procedure, continuous blood pressure and electrocardiographic monitoring is required because of the potential for perforation or arrhythmia. It is important that a pericardiocentesis kit is readily available, and that the operator possesses the ability to rapidly perform an emergency pericardiocentesis in the event of perforation and tamponade. Rarely, emergency surgery is needed either to correct ongoing bleeding from a perforation or to evacuate the pericardium and relieve tamponade if pericardiocentesis is unsuccessful. For this reason, myocardial biopsies should be performed only at institutions that have this capability.

Right ventricular endomyocardial biopsy is readily performed from the right internal jugular vein. A 7 French (Fr) venous sheath is placed in the right internal jugular vein. A slight curve is added to the end of a disposable bioptome by gently bending the distal 10 to 15 cm of the device allowing the operator the ability to steer the catheter through the cardiac chambers and easily redirect the tip. The operator should be aware of the orientation of the bioptome's curve relative to the handle. This provides important knowledge regarding the location of the tip of the biopsy forceps at all times. With the curve of the bioptome facing the patient's right, the closed bioptome is advanced under fluoroscopic guidance through the venous sheath to the right atrium (Fig. 17-1). The catheter is rotated by flipping the bioptome's handle counterclockwise toward the patient's left side causing the curve of the bioptome to face toward the tricuspid valve, facilitating entry of the bioptome into the right ventricle (Fig. 17-2). The bioptome is gently advanced. Fluoroscopic imaging in the left anterior oblique view helps ensure the tip of the biopsy

Table 17-1.　**Recommendations for Endomyocardial Biopsy Based on Expert Consensus**

Class I Recommendations

(Evidence or agreement that the procedure is beneficial, useful, and effective)
1. Unexplained, new-onset heart failure <2 weeks in duration associated with a normal-sized or dilated left ventricle in addition to hemodynamic compromise
2. Unexplained, new-onset heart failure of 2 weeks to 3 months in duration associated with a dilated left ventricle and new ventricular arrhythmias, Mobitz type II second- or third-degree atrioventricular heart block, or failure to respond to medical therapy within 2 weeks

Class II Recommendations

(Conflicting evidence or disagreement about usefulness/efficacy of a procedure)

Class IIa

(Evidence/opinion favor the procedures usefulness/efficacy)
1. Unexplained heart failure >3 months in duration associated with a dilated left ventricle and new ventricular arrhythmias, Mobitz type II second- or third-degree atrioventricular heart block, or failure to respond to medical therapy within 2 weeks
2. Unexplained heart failure associated with a dilated cardiomyopathy of any duration associated with suspected allergic reaction in addition to eosinophilia
3. Unexplained heart failure from suspected anthracycline cardiomyopathy
4. Heart failure associated with unexplained restrictive cardiomyopathy
5. Suspected cardiac tumors where diagnosis cannot be established by imaging modalities
6. Unexplained cardiomyopathy in children

Class IIb

(Little evidence/opinion supporting usefulness/efficacy)
1. Unexplained, new-onset heart failure of 2 weeks to 3 months in duration associated with a dilated left ventricle without ventricular arrhythmias, Mobitz type II second- or third-degree atrioventricular heart block that responds to medical therapy within 2 weeks
2. Unexplained heart failure of >3 months in duration associated with a dilated left ventricle, without new ventricular arrhythmias, Mobitz type II second- or third-degree atrioventricular heart block that responds to medical therapy within 2 weeks
3. Heart failure associated with unexplained hypertrophic cardiomyopathy to search for infiltrative diseases
4. Suspected arrhythmogenic right ventricular dysplasia/cardiomyopathy
5. Unexplained ventricular arrhythmias

Class III Recommendations

(Evidence or opinion that the procedure is not useful or effective and, in some cases, may be harmful)
Unexplained atrial fibrillation

Adapted from Cooper LT, Baughman KL, Feldman AM, et al: American Heart Association. American College of Cardiology. European Society of Cardiology. The role of endomyocardial biopsy in the management of cardiovascular disease: A scientific statement from the American Heart Association, the American College of Cardiology, and the European Society of Cardiology. Circulation 2007;116:2216–2233, by permission.

forceps is directed posteriorly, and thus against the interventricular septum, the safest location to biopsy.

Demonstration of ventricular ectopy ensures that the bioptome has entered the right ventricle. Absence of ventricular ectopy indicates that the bioptome has not yet crossed the tricuspid valve and either remains in the right atrium or the bioptome has inadvertently entered the coronary sinus. Neither location is appropriate or safe for this procedure. A biopsy should never be attempted unless ventricular ectopy has been noted, confirming an intraventricular location. When the operator is convinced that the bioptome is within the right ventricle and against the septum, the forceps are opened and the catheter advanced to apply gentle forward pressure on the biopsy site (Fig. 17-3). Ectopy is again noted. The forceps are closed and withdrawn from the body and the sample collected.

Biopsy from the femoral vein requires the positioning of a long sheath in the right ventricle. After obtaining femoral venous access, a 6 Fr pigtail catheter is inserted into a 7 Fr, 98-cm 40-degree curved sheath and directed to the right atrium using a 0.035-inch J-tipped guide wire (Fig. 17-4). The pigtail catheter is turned toward the tricuspid orifice and the guide wire is advanced across the tricuspid valve (Fig. 17-5). The pigtail catheter is then advanced over the wire and passed into the right ventricle. The wire and pigtail catheter is fixed in this position and the sheath advanced over the pigtail catheter into the right ventricle (Fig. 17-6). The pigtail catheter and guide wire are then removed, leaving the sheath in the right ventricle (Fig. 17-7). The sheath should be allowed to bleed back to expel any air that may have entered the sheath and then gently flushed with heparinized saline. The sheath is manipulated in the left anterior oblique view so that it points toward the septum; ventricular ectopy should again be noted.

It is imperative to achieve satisfactory sheath position within the right ventricle because the bioptome will be directed to the position determined by the sheath. The bioptome is advanced until it exits the distal end of the sheath and the forceps opened (Fig. 17-8). The bioptome is further advanced so that the open jaws come into contact with the endocardial surface, manifest by development of ventricular ectopy. This sometimes requires advancement of the entire sheath. Once the open bioptome is against the myocardium, the jaws are closed, the bioptome retracted from the sheath, and the samples collected.

Ideally, sequential biopsies are obtained from different sites within the right ventricle by changing the position of the bioptome. In reality, this may be difficult to accomplish. Usually, four to five samples are collected with each sample about 1 to 2 mm^3. The biopsy samples should be carefully handled, placed in formalin, and promptly sent to the pathology laboratory for preparation and analysis.

Complications. Endomyocardial biopsy has several important risks. Commonly observed complications are principally related to vascular access. These include access-site bleeding, inadvertent arterial puncture, hematoma, nerve injury, or pneumothorax. Minor complications such as atrial or ventricular arrhythmias, heart block, and vasovagal reactions are self-limited and typically resolve by the time the patient leaves the cardiac catheterization laboratory.

Cardiac perforation leading to bleeding into the pericardial space and cardiac tamponade is the most dreaded and potentially life-threatening complication from a heart biopsy. Fortunately, this problem is rare, accounting for less than 1% of procedures (2). Tamponade rarely complicates biopsy in patients with prior heart transplantation, probably because of the associated scarring and lack of pericardium, preventing tamponade. In addition to transplantation status, other patients at increased risk for perforation and tamponade include those with increased right ventricular systolic pressures, right ventricular dilatation, and patients with platelet dysfunction or coagulopathy. Perforation usually manifests within minutes causing marked hypotension, elevated neck veins, and acute dyspnea. Dramatic cardiovascular collapse may ensue despite the presence of a relatively small effusion. Prompt management with saline boluses and vasopressors help initially resuscitate the patient, but this complication often requires an emergent pericardiocentesis. Echocardiography confirms the diagnosis and helps guide a potentially difficult pericardiocentesis in the event there is only a small volume of blood causing tamponade. Pericardiocentesis quickly improves the hemodynamics. The drain is often left in place to monitor the extent of ongoing bleeding. In most cases, the perforation seals spontaneously. Exceptions include individuals with marked right ventricular hypertension or coagulopathy. Continued bleeding in these situations may require surgical correction of the perforation.

Additional, rare complications include damage to the tricuspid valve and significant tricuspid regurgitation, pacemaker lead dislodgement, and the creation of a fistula from the ventricular chamber to a vein or coronary arteriole (Videos 17-1 and 17-2). The latter finding may be observed in the post-transplant patient who has had multiple biopsy procedures over many years and is usually of no clinical consequence.

References

1. Cooper LT, Baughman KL, Feldman AM, et al: American Heart Association. American College of Cardiology. European Society of Cardiology. The role of endomyocardial biopsy in the management of cardiovascular disease: A scientific statement from the American Heart Association, the American College of Cardiology, and the European Society of Cardiology. Circulation 2007;116:2216–2233.
2. Deckers JW, Hare JM, Baughman KL: Complications of transvenous right ventricular endomyocardial biopsy in adult patients with cardiomyopathy: A seven-year survey of 546 consecutive diagnostic procedures in a tertiary referral center. J Am Coll Cardiol 1992;19:43–47.

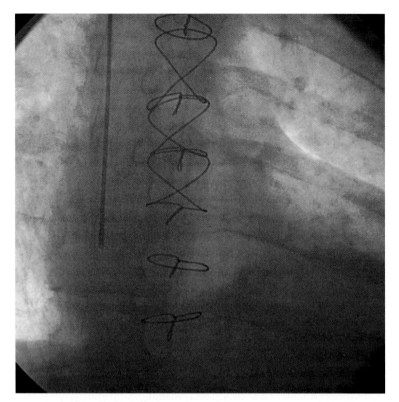

FIGURE 17-1. Technique of endomyocardial biopsy from the right internal jugular vein: The bioptome is advanced into the right atrium.

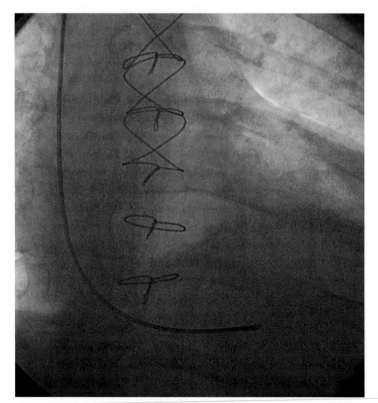

FIGURE 17-2. Technique of endomyocardial biopsy from the right internal jugular vein: The bioptome has been advanced across the tricuspid valve and into the right ventricle.

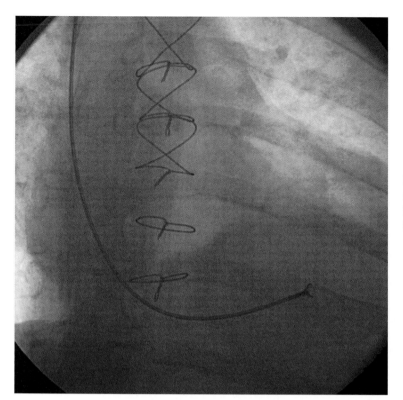

FIGURE 17-3. Technique of endomyocardial biopsy from the right internal jugular vein: The bioptome forceps have been opened and pushed against the right ventricular myocardium.

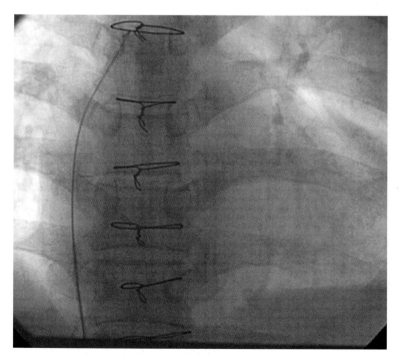

FIGURE 17-4. Technique of endomyocardial biopsy from the right femoral vein: A guide wire is positioned in the superior vena cava, and a long, curved sheath loaded on a pigtail catheter is advanced to the right atrium.

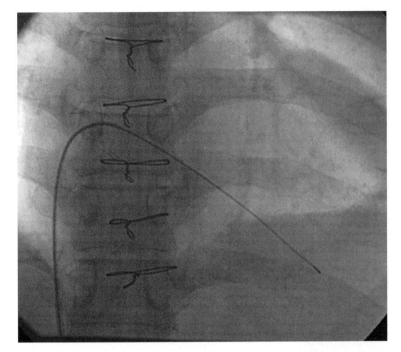

FIGURE 17-5. Technique of endomyocardial biopsy from the right femoral vein: The pigtail catheter is pointed toward the tricuspid valve and the guide wire is passed into the right ventricle.

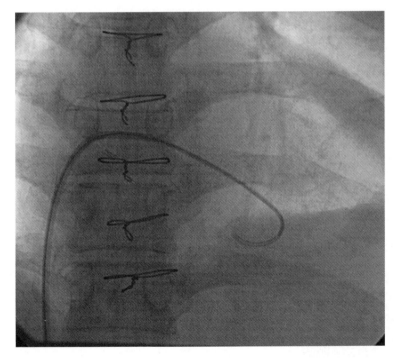

FIGURE 17-6. Technique of endomyocardial biopsy from the right femoral vein: The pigtail catheter is placed into the right ventricle and the guidewire is removed. The long, curved sheath is gently advanced over the pigtail catheter and into the right ventricle.

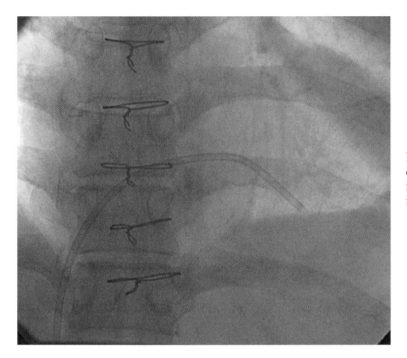

FIGURE 17-7. Technique of endomyocardial biopsy from the right femoral vein: The pigtail catheter is removed with the long, curved sheath remaining in the right ventricle.

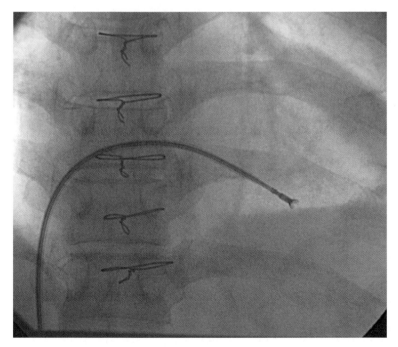

FIGURE 17-8. Technique of endomyocardial biopsy from the right femoral vein: The bioptome is advanced within the sheath. Once the forceps exits the sheath, the bioptome is opened and advanced against the myocardium, and the biopsy is obtained.

CHAPTER 18

EVALUATION OF PROSTHETIC HEART VALVES

For more than 50 years, surgeons have implanted an interesting array of prosthetic heart valves, creating unique challenges to cardiologists when these patients require catheterization. In patients with prosthetic valves, cardiac catheterization may be performed to evaluate suspected prosthetic valve dysfunction, coexisting valvular disease, or the presence of coronary artery disease. Important issues in patients with prosthetic valves undergoing catheterization include the timing and method of interrupting therapeutic anticoagulation, the safety of crossing a prosthetic valve with a catheter, and the recognition of normal and abnormal prosthetic valve function.

Mechanical prosthetic valves require full, systemic anticoagulation with a goal prothrombin time international normalized ratio (INR) of 3.0 to prevent thrombosis or embolism (1). For patients requiring cardiac catheterization, interruption of anticoagulation is necessary to reduce the risk for access-site bleeding. Thus, the clinician must balance the risk for thrombosis with the risk for bleeding, and carefully determine when and how to interrupt and resume anticoagulation. Clinical variables important to this decision include the type of mechanical prosthesis, the position of the valve (aortic versus mitral), left ventricular function, underlying rhythm (sinus vs. atrial fibrillation), and history of prior thromboembolic events. Patients with bileaflet mechanical valves in the aortic position, with normal ventricular function, normal sinus rhythm, and no prior thromboembolic event are at low risk. For patients at low risk, full anticoagulation can be safely suspended for several days. In these cases, warfarin is stopped for 48 to 72 hours and catheterization performed when the INR is less than 1.6. Assuming there are no bleeding concerns related to the procedure, warfarin is resumed 24 hours after catheterization and allowed to increase to the therapeutic level. Patients with mechanical valves in the mitral or tricuspid position, or patients with prosthetic valves in the aortic position with coexisting poor left ventricular function, atrial fibrillation, or a history of prior thromboembolic events are at high risk. For patients at high risk, a "bridging" strategy may be considered. In these cases, warfarin is stopped 48 to 72 hours before the anticipated procedure, and enoxaparin injections or unfractionated heparin infusion is initiated when INR is less than 2.0 to achieve therapeutic systemic anticoagulation until the INR is less than 1.6, at which point enoxaparin or heparin is held for 4 to 6 hours and catheterization performed. After catheterization, oral warfarin is restarted and either enoxaparin or heparin resumed approximately 6 to 12 hours after hemostasis and continued until the INR is therapeutic.

Another important issue relates to the wisdom of passing a catheter across a prosthetic valve. In general, bioprosthetic valves may be treated like native valves and safely crossed with a catheter using the same techniques as for native valves. Mechanical valves, however, cannot be safely crossed. The catheter may become entrapped or may force the valve in an open position causing acute regurgitation and catastrophic hemodynamic collapse. For this reason, if it is important to enter the left ventricle with a catheter in a patient with a mechanical aortic valve, a trans-septal catheterization is often necessary. However, if the operator seeks only hemodynamic information, a 0.014-inch pressure wire can be positioned safely across a mechanical aortic valve providing left ventricular pressure, obviating the need for a trans-septal catheterization (2).

It is crucial for the cardiologist to understand the characteristics of the normally functioning prosthesis and to recognize abnormal valve function. Valve function can be determined in the cardiac catheterization laboratory by integrating the fluoroscopic, hemodynamic, and angiographic findings. Fluoroscopic assessment is a valuable means to rapidly, safely, and inexpensively assess valve function. Hemodynamic measurements obtained in the cardiac catheterization laboratory can precisely measure the degree of obstruction across a prosthetic valve, and these can be compared with the expected degree of stenosis characteristic of the valve make, size, and position. Angiography can quantitate the degree of regurgitation; small degrees of regurgitation may be present normally in some valves but not in others.

Types of Prosthetic Valves. Since the early 1960s, many different mechanical and bioprosthetic valve designs have been engineered and implanted (Table 18-1). Many of these valves are now obsolete and no longer implanted but are still seen in patients today. Each of these has fairly characteristic fluoroscopic appearances (Figs. 18-1 through 18-10). Mechanical St. Jude valves are sometimes particularly difficult to see on fluoroscopy because many of the various iterations of this valve consist of a radiolucent annulus. The thin leaflets are radio-opaque but are nearly invisible in many views. Newer versions of the St. Jude valve have an opaque annular ring. Both the Carpentier–Edwards and Hancock valves are bioprosthetic valves but differ in their appearance; the Hancock valve consists simply of a radio-opaque ring.

Normal Valve Fluoroscopy. In the cardiac catheterization laboratory, prosthetic valve evaluation begins with fluoroscopy. The prosthetic annulus should be assessed for abnormal "rocking" motion indicating partial dehiscence of the valve, usually present when there is endocarditis or a paravalvular leak. For bioprosthetic valves, the leaflets cannot be seen and only the annulus can be evaluated fluoroscopically. Much more information regarding valve function can be learned by fluoroscopy of mechanical valves. The operator can watch the valve open and close, and the normal parameters for these features are well-described for each type of prosthesis. Deviation from these appearances leads one to suspect valve dysfunction.

Table 18-1.	Common Prosthetic Heart Valves

A. Mechanical Valves

1. Caged ball
   Starr–Edwards
   McGovern

2. Single tilting disc
   Björk–Shiley
   Medtronic Hall

3. Bileaflet tilting disc
   St. Jude
   Carbomedics

B. Bioprosthetic Valves

1. Heterograft
   Hancock
   Carpentier–Edwards
   Ionescu–Shiley

2. Homograft

For caged ball prostheses, the ball should freely strike both boundaries of the cage during systole and diastole (Video 18-1). Lack of coaptation of the ball to a portion of the cage or the presence of a gap suggests pannus formation or thrombus in the valve. These valves are clearly seen in almost any radiographic projection; a straight anteroposterior view is often used for the aortic position and 30 degrees right anterior oblique for the mitral position. On aortography (for aortic prostheses) or left ventriculography (for mitral prostheses), there may normally be a small amount (1+) of central regurgitation for caged ball valves (Video 18-2). Degrees of regurgitation greater than this are abnormal and suggest valvular dysfunction or paravalvular leaks.

The various types of tilting disc valves have unique and characteristic appearances on fluoroscopy in the open and closed positions. For example, the leaflets of a St. Jude bileaflet tilting disc valve should appear nearly parallel in the open position, and in the closed position, the leaflets should appear as a "v" with an apex angle between 120 and 130 degrees depending on the size of the valve (Video 18-3). Prosthetic valve dysfunction is present if one of the valve leaflets appears immobile, does not parallel the motion of the other leaflet, or if there is limited excursion of one or both leaflets. Normally functioning tilting disc valves are not associated with any significant degree of regurgitation. Single tilting disc valves also have characteristic open and closed appearances; for example, the disc of the normally functioning Medtronic Hall mechanical prosthesis opens to 75 degrees in the aortic position and 70 degrees in the mitral position (Video 18-4). The fluoroscopic appearance of a normally functioning Björk–Shiley prosthesis is shown in Video 18-5.

Normal Valve Gradients. Depending on the type and size of the prosthesis, all artificial valves obstruct the orifice to some degree. Among the various mechanical prostheses, the caged ball valves are the most obstructive and the bileaflet tilting disc valves are the least; the single tilting disc valves are in between. Among bioprosthetic grafts, porcine heterografts have fairly low profiles compared with mechanical valves with the largest valve areas attributed to homografts. It is important for the cardiologist to know the expected valve gradients of the prosthesis used in his or her patient; these have been reported for a variety of commonly seen valves in both the mitral and the aortic position, and are summarized in Table 18-2 (3). Pressure gradients in excess of these may indicate prosthetic valve dysfunction from pannus formation or patient-prosthesis mismatch (4). As noted earlier, mechanical valves cannot be safely crossed with a catheter. Thus, determining the pressure gradient across a mechanical valve in the aortic position requires simultaneous pressure measurements from a catheter in the aorta and from a catheter placed in the left ventricle via a trans-septal catheterization. Alternatively, a 0.014-inch pressure wire can be safely placed retrograde across a mechanical valve to measure left ventricular pressure. An example of this approach to assess a pressure gradient across a St. Jude valve in the aortic position is shown in Figure 18-11.

Prosthetic Valve Dysfunction. Serious abnormalities affecting prosthetic valves include valve thrombosis, structural deterioration of the valve, and paravalvular leaks.

Valve Thrombosis. Acute thrombosis of a prosthetic valve is a medical emergency. This complication may be seen in up to 5% of mechanical valves and is usually associated with subtherapeutic anticoagulation. Thrombosis rarely affects bioprosthetic valves. Patients usually present with acute pulmonary edema, hypotension, or shock caused by acute valve obstruction or valve regurgitation from a leaflet trapped in the open position by the clot. Embolic events such as stroke, acute myocardial infarction, or acute limb ischemia may also occur. A more indolent or chronic presentation is possible from the slow development of pannus formation on the valve. Diagnosis can be made by echocardiography or, in the cardiac catheterization laboratory, by fluoroscopy. Examples of the fluoroscopic appearance of valve thrombosis are shown in Videos 18-6 and 18-7.

Treatment of valve thrombosis depends on the patient's hemodynamic stability, comorbid illness, suitability for reoperation, as well as the size and acuity of the thrombus (1). Clinicians have to choose between reoperation and lytic therapy; both carry substantial risk, and

Table 18-2.	Expected Doppler Gradients across Common Prostheses		
VALVE	SIZE	MEAN GRADIENT	ORIFICE AREA
Mitral Position			
Starr–Edwards (ball and cage)	28	7 ± 3 mm Hg	1.9 ± 0.6 cm^2
	30	7 ± 3 mm Hg	1.7 ± 0.4 cm^2
	32	5 ± 3 mm Hg	2.0 ± 0.4 cm^2
Björk–Shiley (single tilting disc)	27	5 ± 2 mm Hg	1.8 ± 0.5 cm^2
	29	3 ± 1 mm Hg	2.1 ± 0.4 cm^2
	31	2 ± 2 mm Hg	2.2 ± 0.3 cm^2
St. Jude (bileaflet tilting disc)	27	5 ± 2 mm Hg	1.7 ± 0.2 cm^2
	29	4 ± 2 mm Hg	1.8 ± 0.2 cm^2
	31	4 ± 2 mm Hg	2.0 ± 0.3 cm^2
Carbomedics (bileaflet tilting disc)	25	4 ± 1 mm Hg	2.9 ± 0.8 cm^2
	27	3 ± 1 mm Hg	2.9 ± 0.8 cm^2
	29	3 ± 1 mm Hg	2.3 ± 0.4 cm^2
	31	3 ± 1 mm Hg	2.8 ± 1.0 cm^2
Carpentier Edwards (pericardial)	29	5 ± 2 mm Hg	NA
	31	4 ± 1 mm Hg	NA
Hancock II (porcine)	27	NA	2.2 ± 0.1 cm^2
	29	NA	2.8 ± 0.1 cm^2
	31	NA	2.8 ± 0.1 cm^2
	33	NA	3.2 ± 0.2 cm^2
Aortic Position			
Starr–Edwards (ball and cage)	23	22 ± 9 mm Hg	1.1 cm^2
	24	22 ± 8 mm Hg	NA
	26	20 ± 6 mm Hg	NA
	27	19 ± 4 mm Hg	1.8 cm^2
St. Jude (bileaflet tilting disc)	19	19 ± 6 mm Hg	1.0 ± 0.2 cm^2
	21	16 ± 6 mm Hg	1.3 ± 0.3 cm^2
	23	14 ± 5 mm Hg	1.6 ± 0.4 cm^2
	25	13 ± 5 mm Hg	1.9 ± 0.5 cm^2
	27	11 ± 5 mm Hg	2.4 ± 0.6 cm^2
Carbomedics (bileaflet tilting disc)	19	12 ± 5 mm Hg	1.3 ± 0.4 cm^2
	21	13 ± 4 mm Hg	1.4 ± 0.4 cm^2
	23	11 ± 4 mm Hg	1.7 ± 0.3 cm^2
	25	9 ± 5 mm Hg	2.0 ± 0.4 cm^2
	27	8 ± 3 mm Hg	2.6 ± 0.3 cm^2
Carpentier–Edwards (pericardial)	21	17 ± 6 mm Hg	1.5 ± 0.3 cm^2
	23	16 ± 6 mm Hg	1.7 ± 0.5 cm^2
	25	13 ± 4 mm Hg	1.9 ± 0.5 cm^2
	27	12 ± 6 mm Hg	2.3 ± 0.6 cm^2
Hancock II (porcine)	21	15 ± 4 mm Hg	1.2 ± 0.3 cm^2
	23	17 ± 7 mm Hg	1.4 ± 0.2 cm^2
	25	11 ± 3 mm Hg	1.5 ± 0.2 cm^2

From Rosenhek R, Binder T, Maurer G, Baumgartner H: Normal values for Doppler echocardiographic assessment of heart valve prostheses. J Am Soc Echocardiogr 2003;16:116–127.

the best treatment is controversial and evolving. Patients with significant valve dysfunction and large thrombi on echocardiography who are surgical candidates and patients with subacute or chronic presentation who likely have pannus formation are usually best managed with a reoperation. Lytic therapy is often prescribed for patients who are not surgical candidates. An example of a patient at high risk for reoperation with acute pulmonary edema caused by thrombosis of an aortic prosthesis treated successfully with thrombolytic therapy is shown in Videos 18-8 through 18-10.

Structural Deterioration of a Prosthetic Valve. Current generation mechanical valves are extremely durable and are not prone to structural failure. A notable exception affected an early model of the Björk-Shiley prosthesis (60-degree convexo-concave model) in which catastrophic strut fracture occurred in 1.7 of 1000 valves per year. This valve was removed from the market. However, bioprosthetic valves are prone to structural deterioration over time.

Thrombotic obstruction is rare. Immunologic reactions causing accelerated tissue growth and stenosis may rarely affect some bioprosthesis early after implantation (Video 18-11). Late tissue failure is a more common and well-known limitation of bioprosthetic valves. Calcification, leaflet thickening, leaflet tears, and detachment may occur and cause either stenosis or regurgitation of the valve.

Paravalvular Leaks. Paravalvular leaks result from partial separation of the prosthetic valve sewing ring from the native valve annulus. Small paravalvular leaks are not uncommon and rarely lead to significant sequelae. Large paravalvular leaks are associated with symptoms and consequences from severe regurgitation; they are also associated with hemolysis. The predisposing risk factors for paravalvular leaks include the presence of heavy mitral annular calcification, native valve endocarditis, myxomatous degeneration of the valve, and postoperative, prosthetic valve endocarditis. Fluoroscopy may reveal abnormal rocking motion of the annulus (Video 18-12). The paravalvular leak is usually clearly evident by aortography in the case of an aortic prosthesis (Videos 18-13 and 18-14) and by left ventriculography in the case of a mitral paravalvular leak (Videos 18-15 and 18-16).

References

1. Bonow RO, Carabello BA, Chatterjee K, et al: ACC/AHA 2006 guidelines for the management of patients with valvular heart disease: A report of the American College of Cardiology/American Heart Association Task Force on Practice Guidelines (Writing Committee to Develop Guidelines for the Management of Patients with Valvular Heart Disease). American College of Cardiology Web Site. Available at: http://www.acc.org/clinical/guidelines/valvular/index.pdf.
2. Parham W, El Shafei A, Rajjoub H, et al: Retrograde left ventricular hemodynamic assessment across bileaflet prosthetic aortic valves: The use of a high-fidelity pressure sensor angioplasty guidewire. Catheter Cardiovasc Interv 2003;59:509–513.
3. Rosenhek R, Binder T, Maurer G, Baumgartner H: Normal values for Doppler echocardiographic assessment of heart valve prostheses. J Am Soc Echocardiogr 2003;16:116–127.
4. Ragosta M: Hemodynamic rounds: Determination of the source and severity of a transvalvular left ventricular outflow tract gradient in patients with a prosthetic aortic valve. Catheter Cardiovasc Interv 2007;70:809–814.

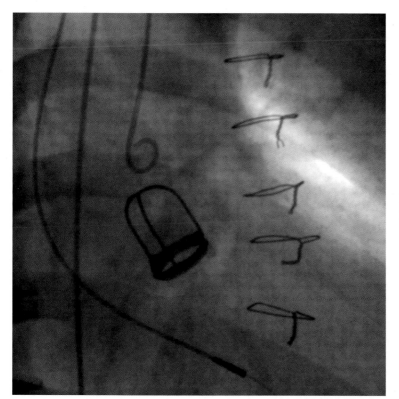

FIGURE 18-1. Example of a caged-ball prosthesis placed in the aortic position (Starr–Edwards valve).

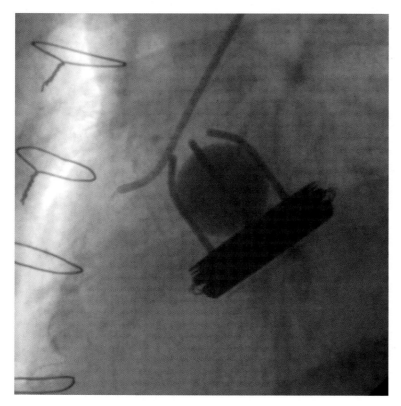

FIGURE 18-2. Example of an archaic caged ball prosthesis placed in the aortic position (Magovern valve).

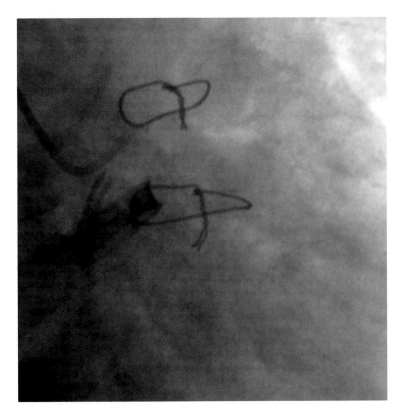

FIGURE 18-3. Characteristic appearance of a Lillehei–Kaster single tilting disc prosthesis with two "horns" on the lateral aspects of the valve.

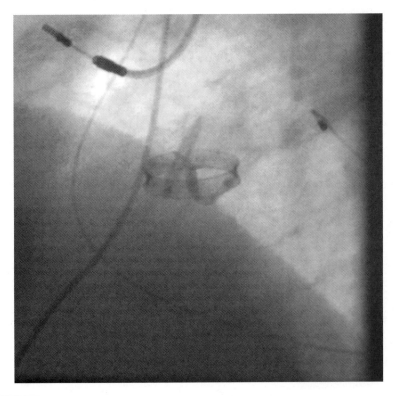

FIGURE 18-4. Example of a Medtronic Hall single tilting disc prosthesis.

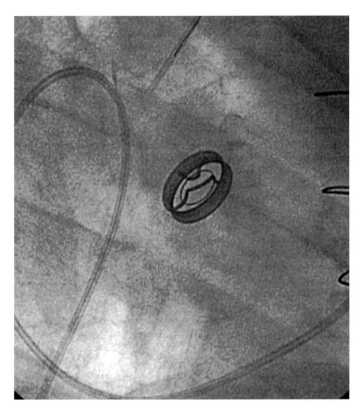

FIGURE 18-5. Example of a Björk–Shiley single tilting disc prosthesis.

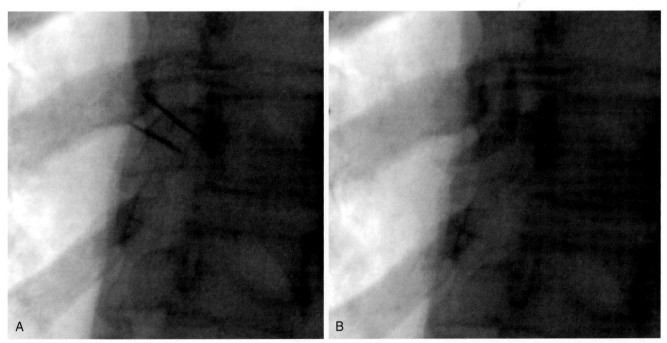

FIGURE 18-6. Example of the St. Jude bileaflet-disc, mechanical prosthesis in the open (A) and closed (B) positions. The annular ring may be transparent (as in this case) or may be densely opaque.

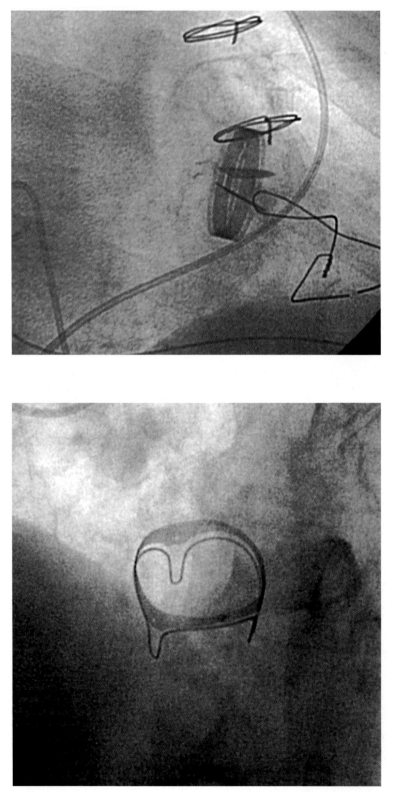

FIGURE 18-7. Another type of bileaflet-disc mechanical valve is shown (ATS valve).

FIGURE 18-8. Example of a bioprosthetic valve (Paramount pericardial valve) in the mitral position.

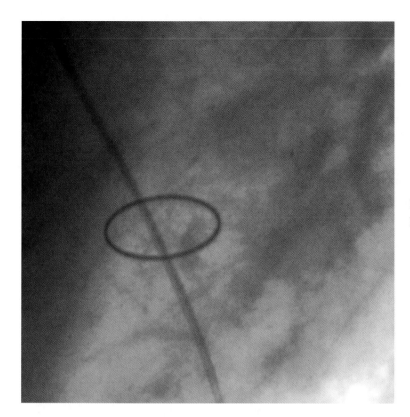

FIGURE 18-9. Example of a Hancock porcine prosthesis.

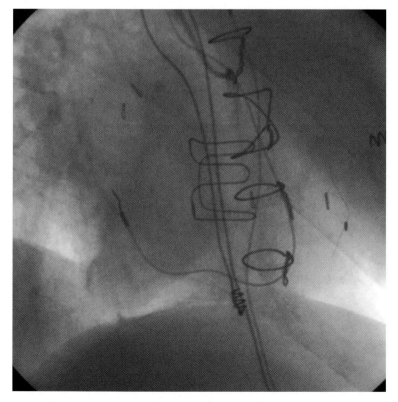

FIGURE 18-10. Carpentier–Edwards bioprosthetic valve.

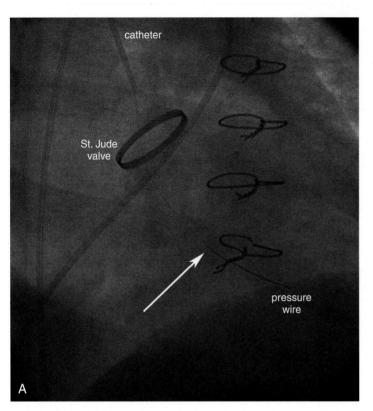

A

FIGURE 18-11. The use of a pressure wire technique to assess the pressure gradient across a mechanical aortic valve prosthesis is shown. *A,* A multipurpose catheter is positioned above a St. Jude bileaflet tilting disc valve with the pressure wire advanced across the valve leaflets into the left ventricle. *Arrow* indicates the pressure transducer. This arrangement allows simultaneous aortic and left ventricular pressure measurement

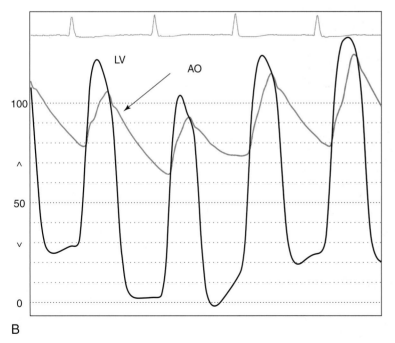

B

FIGURE 18-11. cont'd *(B).* The observed pressure gradient is within the range expected for this size and type of prosthesis.